STUDY GUIDE TO ACCOMPANY

Respiratory Care Equipment

STUDY GUIDE TO ACCOMPANY
Respiratory Care Equipment

Mark L. Simmons, MSEd, RPFT, RRT

Director, School of Respiratory Care
York Hospital
York College of Pennsylvania
York, Pennsylvania

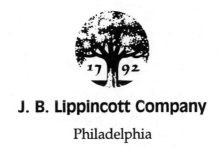

J. B. Lippincott Company

Philadelphia

Sponsoring Editor: Andrew Allen
Coordinating Editorial Assistant: Laura Dover
Cover Designer: Lou Fuiano
Production Manager: Virginia Barishek
Composition and Production: Till & Till, Inc.
Printer/Binder: Capital City Press
Cover Printer: Lehigh Press

6 5 4 3 2 1

(∞) This paper meets the requirements of ANSI/NISO Z39.48-1992 (permanence of paper).

Any procedure or practice described in this book should be applied by the health care practitioner under appropriate supervision in accordance with professional standards of care used with regard to the unique circumstances that apply in each practice situation. Care has been taken to confirm the accuracy of information presented and to describe generally accepted practices. However, the authors, editors, and publisher cannot accept any responsibility for errors or omissions or for any consequences from application of the information in this book and make no warranty, express or implied, with respect to the contents of the book.

Every effort has been made to ensure drug selections and dosages are in accordance with current recommendations and practice. Because of ongoing research, changes in government regulations and the constant flow of information on drug therapy, reactions and interactions, the reader is cautioned to check the package insert for each drug for indications, dosages, warnings and precautions, particularly if the drug is new or infrequently used.

*This study guide is dedicated to the many students
with whom I have had the privilege of sharing respiratory care
during my 18-year career.
They have richly enhanced my life.*

Preface

This study guide is designed primarily for students using *Respiratory Care Equipment* by Branson, Hess, and Chatburn. However, it may also serve as a worthwhile tool for respiratory care practitioners who wish to review or update their skills. The workbook parallels *Respiratory Care Equipment*. It is intended to provide a practical and useful highlight of topics and information that are most important or most often require review. Along with the discussion of topics, there are several types of exercises included in the study guide. These include: mathematical calculations, clinical problem solving, critical thinking exercises, laboratory exercises, possible research projects, review (multiple choice) questions, and suggested field trips. A few notes of importance should be listed concerning these exercises.

- Not all types of exercises are found in all chapters. They were developed as appropriate based on the chapter content and the information presented.
- The laboratory exercises may require instructor guidance.
- Answers given to the clinical problem solving and critical thinking exercises are not necessarily the only possible solutions.
- Although the term "trouble-shooting" is not used in the text headings, many of the exercises incorporate trouble-shooting skills.
- The answers to the various exercises can be found at the back of the text.

I believe this study guide will be a good companion to *Respiratory Care Equipment*. I believe it will also enhance the student's learning process when studying respiratory care equipment.

Mark L. Simmons, MSEd, RPFT, RRT

Acknowledgments

Deep gratitude is expressed to:

Christopher Furtaw, BS, RRT, for his review of the text, and his role in generating the answers for the answer key.

Priscilla Simmons, EdD, RN, my wife, for her proofreading, her valuable suggestions, and her encouragement throughout the project.

My sons, Clinton and Teddy, for their patience when dad was unavailable to play games.

Contents

1

Physical Properties of Gases and Principles of Gas Movement

INTRODUCTION

All matter exists in three states: solid, liquid, and gas. This chapter deals with gases and the factors affecting them.

TEMPERATURE SCALES

Three temperature scales are routinely used in clinical practice and for calculation of pressure and volume changes. These are the Fahrenheit (F), Celsius (C), and Kelvin (K) scales. To convert from one temperature scale to another the following formulas are used:

$$C = (F - 32)\, \tfrac{5}{9}$$

$$F = \tfrac{9}{5}C + 32$$

$$K = C + 273 \;\; \text{(Absolute temperature scale)}$$

Temperature Conversions: Student Exercise

Perform the following temperature conversions.

1-1.   37°C to F   _____

1-2.   60°C to F   _____

1-3.   –20°C to F   _____

1-4.   212°F to C   _____

1-5.   0°F to C   _____

1-6.   –40°F to C   _____

1-7.   10°C to K   _____

1-8.   50°C to K   _____

1-9.   –60°C to K   _____

1-10.   0°K to C   _____

1-11.   150°K to C   _____

1-12.   350°K to C   _____

1-13.   273°K to F   _____

1-14.   310°K to F   _____

1-15.   100°K to F   _____

1-16.   373°F to °K   _____

1-17.   24°F to °K   _____

1-18.   –100°F to °K   _____

PRESSURE MEASUREMENTS

The pressure exerted by a gas is affected by the number of molecules present, the temperature of the system, and the volume of the container. Pressure can be measured by different methods and can be expressed in a variety of units as atmospheric, gauge, or absolute pressure. Atmospheric pressure (P_{atm}) is the pressure exerted by the atmosphere and is measured with a barometer. Gauge pressure (P_{ga}) is a pressure relative to P_{atm} and is measured using a manometer. At 1 atmospheric pressure, gauge pressure is zero. Absolute pressure (P_{abs}), or total pressure, is the sum of gauge pressure and atmospheric pressure, and is expressed in the following formula:

Absolute pressure = atmospheric pressure + gauge pressure

$$P_{abs} = P_{atm} + P_{ga}$$

TABLE 1-1. Common Values and Units Used to Indicate 1 P_{atm} at Sea Level
760 mm Hg
760 torr
76 cm Hg
1034 cm H_2O
33.9 ft fresh water
33 ft salt water
14.7 psi
29.9 in Hg
101.3 kPa (Kilopascal)
1.014×10^6 dynes/cm^2
1014 millibars
1034 g/cm^2

Pressure is force per unit surface area, yet force and nonforce units are often used to indicate pressure. Examples of force units include: psi, dynes/cm^2, and g/cm^2. Examples of nonforce units include: mm Hg, cm H_2O, and ft H_2O. It is commonly accepted to indicate pressure in the units of the height of a column of fluid since the column will result in a pressure. Many of the commonly used measurements to indicate 1 P_{atm} are listed in Table 1-1.

Since each of the values listed in Table 1-1 is equal to 1 P_{atm}, each is also equal to the others. Conversion from one unit to another can easily be made by using the factors from the conversion chart (Table 1-1 in *Respiratory Care Equipment*) or the formula shown in the following examples, which can be used for conversions between any units.

Examples

Example A: Convert 400 mm Hg to cm H_2O.
- Place the known values for 1 P_{atm} with the appropriate units in the numerators, in this case 760 mm Hg and 1034 cm H_2O.
- Place the given value (400 mm Hg) in the denominator and the unknown value in the other denominator.
- Solve for X. (The values could be rearrange; just be consistent when placing them.)

$$\frac{760 \text{ mm Hg}}{400 \text{ mm Hg}} = \frac{1034 \text{ cm } H_2O}{X \text{ cm } H_2O} \qquad X \text{ cm } H_2O = 544$$

Example B: Convert 12 psi to ft H_2O.

$$\frac{14.7 \text{ psi}}{12.0 \text{ psi}} = \frac{33.9 \text{ ft } H_2O}{X \text{ ft } H_2O} \qquad X \text{ ft } H_2O = 27.7$$

Example C: Convert 37.5 in Hg to P_{atm}.

$$\frac{29.9 \text{ in Hg}}{37.5 \text{ in Hg}} = \frac{1 \text{ } P_{atm}}{X \text{ } P_{atm}} \qquad X \text{ } P_{atm} = 1.25$$

Pressure Conversions: Student Exercise

Perform the following pressure conversions. Try using both the conversion chart and the method shown above.

1-19. 750 mm Hg to in Hg   _____

1-20. 750 mm Hg to cm H_2O _____

1-21. 14 psi to mm Hg   _____

1-22. 14 psi to cm H_2O (fresh)   _____

1-23. 40 ft H_2O (fresh) to atms   _____

1-24. 10 kPa to mm Hg   _____

1-25. 10 kPa to cm H_2O _____

1-26. 40 mm Hg to kPa   _____

1-27. 100 cm H_2O (fresh) to kPa   _____

1-28. 2.5 atmospheres to ft H_2O (salt)   _____

GAS LAWS

The temperature, pressure, and volume of a gas are interrelated. This relationship can be expressed in the following gas laws.

BOYLE'S LAW

At a constant temperature (T), absolute pressure (P) exerted by a gas increases as the volume (V) decreases and vice versa. This relationship is expressed in the following formula:

$$P \times V = \text{a constant}$$

When starting with a given set of conditions (P_1, V_1) and then making a change in pressure or volume, but keeping temperature constant, determine the new pressure and volume values (P_2, V_2) from the following formula:

$$P_1 \times V_1 = P_2 \times V_2$$

Remember that pressure must be expressed as absolute pressure. If the final answer is to be expressed in gauge pressure, P_2 will need to be converted appropriately.

CHARLES' LAW

At a constant pressure (P), as volume (V) increases, absolute temperature (T) increases and vice versa. This relationship can be expressed in the following formula:

$$V/T = a \text{ constant}$$

When starting with a given set of conditions (V_1, T_1) and then making a change in volume or temperature, but keeping pressure constant, determine the new volume and temperature values (V_2, T_2) from the following formula:

$$V_1/T_1 = V_2/T_2$$

Remember that temperature must be expressed in the absolute temperature scale of Kelvin. If the final answer is to be expressed in Celsius or Fahrenheit, T_2 must be converted back to the appropriate temperature scale.

GAY–LUSSAC'S LAW

At a constant volume (V), as absolute temperature (T) increases, absolute pressure (P) increases and vice versa. This relationship can be expressed in the following formula:

$$P/T = a \text{ constant}$$

When starting with a given set of conditions (P_1, T_1) and then making a change in pressure or temperature, but keeping volume constant, determine the new pressure and temperature values (P_2, T_2) from the following formula:

$$P_1/T_1 = P_2/T_2$$

Remember that both pressure and temperature must be expressed as absolute values in the formula.

COMBINED GAS LAW

The combined gas law places all three variables together in the following formula:

$$P_1 \times V_1/T_1 = P_2 \times V_2/T_2$$

Note that the previous discussion is only valid for dry gases, when relative humidity (RH) equals zero. The formula will need to be modified if water vapor is present. This will be discussed in Chapter 5.

Pressure, Temperature, and Volume Calculations: Student Exercise

Perform the following calculations based on the appropriate gas laws.

- Assume atmospheric pressure of 760 mm Hg if none is given.
- Make sure absolute pressure and temperature are used in the calculations. If a final answer is to be expressed as gauge pressure, P_2 must be converted back to gauge pressure by using the following formula:

$$P_2 - \text{atmospheric pressure} = \text{gauge pressure}$$

Remember to use the same units throughout the problem.

1-29. The gauge pressure of a gas is 50 mm Hg at 0°C. If the volume remains constant, what will the gauge pressure be if the gas is heated to 15°C?

1-30. The gauge pressure of the gas in a full O_2 cylinder is 2200 psi (psig) at 70°F. If volume remains constant, what will the psig of the tank be if the tank is cooled to 30°F?

1-31. A volume of 500 mL is measured at 40°C. If the pressure remains constant, what will the volume be if the temperature decreases to 20°C?

1-32. A volume of 800 mL is measured at 24°C. If pressure remains constant, what will the volume be if the temperature is raised to 37°C?

1-33. The volume of a gas at 770 mm Hg absolute pressure is 1.5 L. If temperature remains constant, what is the volume of the gas at 630 mm Hg absolute pressure?

1-34. The volume of a gas at 0 mm Hg gauge pressure is 2.4 L. What is the gauge pressure if the volume decreases to 2.0 L and the temperature remains constant ?

1-35. For a given system, the initial pressure is 50 cm H_2O (gauge), the temperature is 20°C, and the volume is 1000 mL. What is the final gauge pressure if the temperature climbs to 30°C and the volume is reduced to 900 mL?

1-36. What is the resultant temperature of a system, where the initial pressure is 10 psig, the temperature is 37°C, and the volume is 300 mL, when the pressure drops to 5 psig and the volume increases to 400 mL?

DALTON'S LAW

The total pressure (P_t) of a mixture of gases is equal to the sum of the pressures exerted by each of the individual gases, known as their partial pressures (P_{gas}). The formula expressing this relationship is

$$P_t = P_{gas\,a} + P_{gas\,b} + P_{gas\,c} + \cdots + P_{gas\,n}$$

FRACTIONAL CONCENTRATION OF GAS

Another concept related to this discussion is fractional concentration of gas (F_{gas}). Room air contains approximately 21% O_2 ($FO_2 = .21$) and 79% N_2 ($FN_2 = .79$). To determine the partial pressure exerted by a gas, when the fractional concentration is known, use the following formula:

$$P_t \times F_{gas} = P_{gas}$$

Example
Given $P_{atm} = 760$ mm Hg, $FO_2 = .21$ and $FN_2 = .79$

$$760 \text{ mm Hg} \times .21 = 160 \text{ mm Hg } (PO_2)$$

and

$$760 \text{ mm Hg} \times .79 = 600 \text{ mm Hg } (PN_2)$$

This partial pressure of oxygen is actually the pressure of inspired oxygen and is designated as P_{IO_2}. The P_{N_2} is the pressure of inspired nitrogen and is designated as P_{IN_2}. Using Dalton's law, $P_t = 160$ mm Hg $+ 600$ mm Hg $= 760$ mm Hg.

DETERMINATION OF F$_{gas}$

The F_{gas} can be determined if the P_t and P_{gas} are known by using the following formula:

$$P_{gas}/P_t = F_{gas}$$

Example

160 mm Hg (P_{O_2})/760 mm Hg (P_t) = .21 (F_{O_2}) or 21% O_2 (where $F_{gas} \times 100 = \%$ gas)

Partial Pressure and Percent Calculations: Student Exercise

1-37. Calculate the partial pressure of O_2 (P_{O_2}) and N_2 (P_{N_2}) in a 40%/60% O_2/N_2 mixture, where the total pressure (P_t) is 750 mm Hg.

1-38. Calculate the P_{He} and P_{O_2} in a 80%/20% He/O_2 gas mixture, where the P_t is 770 mm Hg.

1-39. Calculate P_t, F_{O_2}, %O_2, F_{CO_2}, %CO_2, F_{N_2}, and %N_2, if P_{O_2} is 80 mm Hg, P_{CO_2} is 40 mm Hg and P_{N_2} is 500 mm Hg.

1-40. If 100% O_2 is being delivered to a patient and the P_t is 760, what is the P_{O_2}?

HENRY'S LAW

Henry's law is important for allowing the determination of the amount of O_2 dissolved in blood. Clinically the following solubility coefficient is used for O_2:

0.003 mL of O_2/dL of blood/mm Hg   (where dL = deciliter = 100 mL)

Examples

The following examples illustrate how this factor is used to determine the amount of O_2 dissolved in the blood.

Example A: Po2 = 1 mm Hg

$$1 \text{ mm Hg} \times 0.003 \text{ mL } O_2/dL/\text{mm Hg} = 0.003 \text{ mL } O_2/dL$$

Example B: Po2 = 100 mm Hg

$$100 \text{ mm Hg} \times 0.003 \text{ mL } O_2/dL/\text{mm Hg} = 0.3 \text{ mL } O_2/dL$$

Example C: Po2 = 1000 mm Hg

$$1000 \text{ mm Hg} \times 0.003 \text{ mL } O_2/dL/\text{mm Hg} = 3.0 \text{ mL } O_2/dL$$

Note: Example B is a "normal" Po_2, and Example C is an example of a Po_2 under hyperbaric conditions. This will be further discussed in Chapter 4.

Dissolved Oxygen Content Calculations: Student Exercise

Calculate the amount of O_2 dissolved in blood for the following Po_2 values:

	Po_2 (mm Hg)	O_2 Dissolved (mL/dL blood)
1-41.	55	_____
1-42.	80	_____
1-43.	120	_____
1-44.	225	_____
1-45.	600	_____

GAS MIXING

Gas mixing allows the clinician to deliver precise O_2 concentrations to patients by mixing varying amounts of air and O_2. Routinely, room air (21% O_2) and 100% O_2 are the two gases mixed although others could also be mixed. A calculation of FIO_2 can be done when mixing any proportions of air and O_2. The formula is

$$V_1 \times C_1 + V_2 \times C_2 = V_t \times C_t$$

where
   V_1 is the volume of room air
   C_1 is the FO_2 in room air (.21)
   V_2 is the volume of O_2
   C_2 is the FO_2 of 100% O_2 (1.0);
   V_t is the total volume of the mixture
   C_t is the final concentration of the mixture

Example
    7 L of air is mixed with 3 L of O_2

$$7 \times .21 + 3 \times 1 = 10 \times C_t$$

$$(1.47 + 3)/10 = C_t$$

$$C_t = .447 \text{ or } 45\% \ O_2$$

Oxygen Percent Calculations: Student Exercise

Calculate the percent O_2 which results from mixing the following amounts of air and O_2.

Mixtures	O_2 Percent
1-46. 20 L of air and 20 L of O_2	_____
1-47. 5 L of air and 5 L of O_2	_____
1-48. 13 L of air and 2 L of O_2	_____
1-49. 7 L of air and 12 L of O_2	_____
1-50. 21 L of air and 32 L of O_2	_____

ENTRAINMENT

Entrainment (or jet mixing) devices "entrain" room air at a preset ratio determined by the size of the entrainment port (or window) and the size of the jet. To determine the ratio for any given FO_2, the V_1C_1 formula can be used or the "X method" can be utilized.

Example: V_1C_1 Formula
Determine the ratio of air to O_2 (A : O_2) for 40% O_2.

$$V_1 \times C_1 + V_2 \times C_2 = V_t \times C_t$$

To determine ratios, always allow V_2 (the volume of O_2) to equal 1.

$$Z \times .21 + 1 \times 1 = (Z + 1) \times .4$$
$$21Z + 1 = .4Z + .4:$$
$$.6 = .19Z:$$
$$Z = 3.16$$

The A : O_2 ratio for 40% O_2 is approximately 3 : 1.

Example: The "X Method"
Determine the A: O_2 ratio for 40% O_2 by using the "X method" (Figure 1-1).

1. Place the desired O_2 percent in the middle of the X.
2. Place 21 (21% O_2) in the left upper arm of the X.
3. Place 100 (100% O_2) in the left lower leg of the X.
4. Now, following the X pattern, subtract, placing the differences in the right-sided arm and leg. (Keep all numbers positive.)

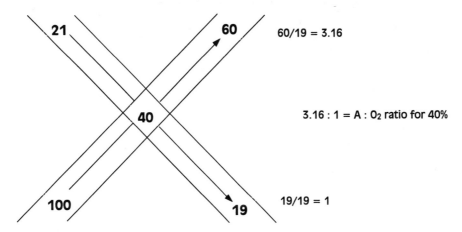

Figure 1-1

5. Divide the value in the right lower leg into both the right upper arm and the right lower leg. This always makes the O_2 value 1.
6. The result of the right upper arm : right lower leg ratio is the A : O_2 ratio for the O_2% in the middle of the X.

Either method is accurate for determining the A : O_2 ratio for any FO_2, although rounding off (room air = 21%, etc.), regardless of the method used, can make the numbers slightly inaccurate. Some of the common ratios are listed in Table 1-2.

TABLE 1-2. A : O_2 Ratios for Common F_{IO_2}s			
A	*O_2*	*Actual O_2 %*	*Commonly Stated O_2 %*
0.6	1	70.4	70
1.0	1	60.5	60
2.0	1	47.3	47
3.0	1	40.7	40
4.0	1	36.8	37
5.0	1	34.2	35
10.0	1	28.2	28
25.0	1	24.0	24

Air : Oxygen Ratio Calculations: Student Exercise

Calculate the ratios for the following F_{IO_2}s. Try using both methods. For consistency, always make O_2 a value of one (1) in the ratio.

	O_2 Percent	$A : O_2$
1-51.	24%	_____
1-52.	26%	_____
1-53.	30%	_____
1-54.	34%	_____
1-55.	55%	_____
1-56.	80%	_____

REVIEW QUESTIONS

1-57. According to the law of continuity, if total flow remains constant, what will happen to velocity if cross-sectional area increases?
  A. not change
  B. increase
  C. decrease

1-58. Normal barometric pressure at sea level can be expressed as:
   I. 14.7 psi
   II. 76 cm Hg
   III. 29.9 ft H_2O
   IV. 760 mm H_2O
  A. I only
  B. I and II only
  C. I, II, and III only
  D. I, III, and IV only

1-59. According to Poiseuille's law, if the length of a tube is decreased, flow through the tube will _____, if all other factors remain constant.
  A. not change
  B. increase
  C. decrease

1-60. Which gas law states that P is inversely related to V?
  A. Boyle's
  B. Charles'
  C. Gay-Lussac's
  D. Dalton's

1-61. Diffusion of gases through a membrane will depend on
  A. the gas concentration gradient across the membrane
  B. thickness of the membrane
  C. surface area of the membrane
  D. all of the above
  E. A and B only

1-62. Which of the gas laws states that P is directly related to T?
  A. Boyle's
  B. Charles'
  C. Gay-Lussac's
  D. Dalton's

1-63. A Reynolds number less than 2000 indicates:
  A. decreased diffusion rates
  B. an increase solubility coefficient
  C. laminar flow
  D. increased resistance

1-64. When gas is released into a vacuum
  A. the volume of the gas rapidly decreases
  B. the pressure of the gas rapidly increases
  C. the temperature of the gas rapidly decreases
  D. all of the above
  E. A and B only

1-65. Gas density has an effect under which of the following flow conditions?
  A. laminar
  B. turbulent
  C. neither A or B
  D. both A and B

1-66. The absence of molecular motion occurs at
  A. the freezing point of water (0°C)
  B. the freezing point of oxygen (–218°C)
  C. the freezing point of hydrogen (–259°C)
  D. absolute zero (–273°C)

1-67. Factors that affect airflow resistance through a tube would include which of the following?
        I. internal diameter
       II. external diameter
      III. length
       IV. wall thickness
  A. I only
  B. I and III only
  C. I, II, and III only
  D. II, III, and IV only

2

Compressed Gases: Manufacture, Storage, and Piping Systems

INTRODUCTION

The handling of medical gases, especially oxygen delivery to patients, has been one of the duties performed by respiratory care practitioners (RCPs) for many years. Although most RCPs today are not responsible for the maintenance or repair of oxygen delivery systems or tanks, it is important to understand the basic operation of the systems. This is necessary so trouble shooting can be performed, proper operation can be assessed, and appropriate patient care can be given. Chapter 2 discusses liquid oxygen systems, both large and small, compressed gas tanks, and air compressors.

GAS CYLINDERS

Although the actual pressures and resultant number of liters of gas for a given cylinder size may vary slightly from manufacturer to manufacturer, the values that will be used for the discussion of oxygen cylinders are listed in Table 2-1.

The values for full cylinders should be memorized (it saves carrying a lot of notes around). The volume of a full cylinder can be expressed in cubic feet, gallons, liters (L), or any other volume expression. Since liters are the most commonly used form of expression,

TABLE 2-1. Common Cylinder Sizes along with Their Filling Volumes and Pressures for Full Cylinders, and the Cylinder Factors			
Cylinder Size	Liters (L)	Pressure (psig)	Factor (L/psig)
D	360	2200	0.16
E	620	2200	0.28
F (M)	3000	2200	1.36
G	5300	2200	2.41
H (K)	6900	2200	3.14

especially when it comes oxygen delivery to patients, it is probably best to memorize the liter values. Since tanks have a relatively small, limited volume of gas available for use, the user should know how to calculate the length of time a cylinder will deliver the appropriate flow of oxygen. The volumes for full cylinders are already listed but there are two ways to determine the actual volume of partially filled cylinders. One is by using the cylinder factor, the other is by setting up a mathematical relationship. The cylinder factor is considered first. This factor is determined by dividing the volume of a full tank by the pressure of a full tank.

Example: Determination of the Cylinder Factor
A full E-cylinder contains 620 L at a pressure of 2200 psig.

$$620 \text{ L}/2200 \text{ psig} = 0.28 \text{ L}/\text{psig}$$

For every one psig generated, there will be 0.28 L of gas in the tank. This value is relatively constant from 0 to 2200 psig and can be used to determine tank contents in L at any pressure.

Example: Determination of Tank Contents Using the Cylinder Factor
An E-cylinder at 2200 psig will contain 620 L of oxygen.

$$2200 \times 0.28 = 620, \text{ a full cylinder}$$

An E-cylinder at 1000 psig will contain 280 L of oxygen.

$$1000 \times 0.28 = 280$$

If a practitioner does not want to memorize the cylinder factors, or to calculate them each time a volume determination must be made, the second method using the following mathematical relationship can be used:

$$\frac{\text{volume of full cylinder}}{\text{pressure of full cylinder}} = \frac{\text{volume of partially full cylinder}}{\text{pressure of partially full cylinder}}$$

Example
An E-cylinder has a pressure of 1000 psig. How many liters are present?

$$\frac{620 \text{ L}}{2200 \text{ psig}} = \frac{X}{2200 \text{ psig}} \qquad X = 282 \text{ L}$$

When comparing the two methods, a slightly different value may result since the value of 0.28 and the other tank factors are rounded off. This process will work for any size gaseous tank. (Make sure the correct values are used for the cylinder in question.)

Once the cylinder contents are known, the duration of time it may be used can be calculated if the flow rate being utilized is also known. The E-cylinder in the previous example contains 280 L. If oxygen is being used at 4 L/min, the cylinder will last for 70 minutes (280 L ÷ 4 L/min = 70 min). Obviously, a full tank should be on standby for use when the one being used runs low. All Respiratory Care departments should have a protocol for changing cylinders.

Note that cylinders delivering oxygen via a regulator set at 50 psig will deliver flow until the cylinder is empty (0 psig). The regulator prevents outlet pressure from going above 50 psig but not below 50 psig. (Refer to Chapter 3.) However, once the pressure is less than 50 psig, equipment attached to the regulator and calibrated to operate at 50 psig (Thorpe tube flowmeters, etc.) will not be accurate in their readings or function properly. It is best, therefore, not to use oxygen cylinders at pressure levels ≤50 psig, but replace them before they reach a pressure of 50 psig. Clearly, waiting to change the tank when it is at 50 psig leaves only a few liters of gas available for use. *Don't* wait that long.

Cylinder Contents and Time of Use Calculations: Student Exercise

For each of the following situations, determine the volume of oxygen contained in the cylinders and the maximum time period for which they can be used. (Compare both methods for determining the cylinder contents.)

	Cylinder Size	psig	Liter Flow	Cylinder Volume	Time Period
2-1.	E	1500	6 L/min	_____	_____
2-2.	E	50	3 L/min	_____	_____
2-3.	D	500	4 L/min	_____	_____
2-4.	D	1200	10 L/min	_____	_____
2-5.	H	1800	5 L/min	_____	_____
2-6.	H	800	2 L/min	_____	_____

Tank Pressure Calculations: Student Exercise

Using the same formulas, although rearranged, calculate the pressure in the following cylinders when the volume is known. Both methods can be used.

	Cylinder Size	Liters	Cylinder Pressure
2-7.	G	1800	_____
2-8.	H (K)	5000	_____
2-9.	F (M)	1000	_____
2-10.	D	100	_____
2-11.	E	400	_____

Clinical Problem Solving

2-12. How many H-cylinders would it take to supply the oxygen needed for continuous use to a home patient who is receiving two L/min for one full week?

2-13. How long will an E-cylinder last during the transport of a patient on a portable mechanical ventilator where the ventilator is set at a tidal volume of 1000 mL, the actual frequency is 10 breaths/min, the inspiratory time is one second, and flow rate is set at 60 L/min? (Assume oxygen is not used for any ventilator functions except for volume delivery.)

Laboratory Exercises

2-14. Obtain several gas cylinders of different sizes and gas contents and perform the following:
   a. Compare the color codes for the different gases.
   b. Identify the markings on the cylinders.
   c. Read the label attached to the cylinder.
   d. Safely transport both a small and large cylinder using the appropriate transport carts.
   e. Compare the design of the tank valve outlets on both a small and large cylinder. What safety systems are present and how do they differ for different gases?
   f. Locate the pressure release devices on both small and large cylinders.

2-15. Using a Bourdon pressure gauge, measure the pressure in the oxygen and air lines delivering pressure to a station outlet.

2-16. "Crack" a cylinder by slowly opening the cylinder valve. Why is this done?

LIQUID OXYGEN

Liquid oxygen changes to gaseous oxygen when it reaches its boiling point. At 1 P_{atm} this occurs at approximately –183°C. This temperature varies depending on the pressure in the system. This phenomenon of liquid turning to gas takes place in both large bulk oxygen delivery systems for hospitals and in small portable systems for individual patient use. One cubic foot equals 28.3 L (this applies to gas or liquid volume). One liter of liquid oxygen weighs 2.5 pounds, and 1 L of liquid oxygen will "evaporate" to become 860 L of gaseous oxygen.

Clinical Problem Solving

Using the above information, calculate the following:

2-17. Three pounds of liquid oxygen in a portable unit will last what maximum time if a patient is using a continuous flow of 2 L/min?

2-18. How many pounds of liquid oxygen will be used in a week by a home patient using 4 L/min continuously?

2-19. How many H-cylinders would be needed to equal the gas volume of a hospital's liquid system which contains 100 cubic feet of liquid oxygen?

Laboratory Exercises

Obtain a liquid oxygen reservoir system for home use and perform the following exercises:

2-20. Document the percent oxygen delivery by analyzing the gas coming from the device at different flow rates.

2-21. Using a manometer, check the operating pressure of the system by connecting it to the outlet port of the unit.

2-22. Using a flow measuring device, document accurate flow rates by measuring the flow delivered by the unit. *Note:* A "normal" flowmeter calibrated to 50 psig cannot be used for accurate flow delivery when operating pressures are less than 50 psig. This will be further discussed in Chapter 3.

Field Trips

2-23. *Local:* Locate the liquid oxygen tank at your institution and identify the following: the liquid storage tank, the vaporizer coils, the back-up system and indicator gauges. Is its location appropriate in relation to nearby structures? Locate the area inside the institution where the pipes enter. Identify the main delivery pipe, the main shut-off valve, and some zone valves located throughout the institution.

2-24. *Extended:* Drive to and tour a liquid oxygen processing plant and/or a tank manufacturer.

OXYGEN CONCENTRATORS

Oxygen concentrators have the ability to separate oxygen from the other gases in the atmosphere and deliver it to patients in concentrations greater than 21%. The molecular sieve type concentrator delivers high concentrations of oxygen—86% to 97%, depending on flow rate utilized. The permeable membrane or enricher type concentrator delivers approximately 40% oxygen at various flow rates.

Laboratory Exercises

Obtain both types of oxygen concentrators and perform the following exercises:

2-25. Document the percent oxygen delivery by analyzing the gas coming from the device at different flow rates.

2-26. Using a manometer, check the operating pressure of the system by connecting it to the outlet port of the unit.

2-27. Using a flow measuring device, document accurate flow rates by measuring the flow delivered by the unit. *Note:* A "normal" flowmeter calibrated to 50 psig cannot be used for accurate flow delivery when operating pressures are less than 50 psig. This will be further discussed in Chapter 3.

AIR COMPRESSORS

The compressed air used in a hospital or home setting can be supplied from tanks but is more frequently supplied by electrical compressors. Compressors are one of three types: diaphragm, piston, or rotary. The small portable compressors used to deliver low flows and/or pressures are usually diaphragm compressors. Piston and rotary compressors are used when high flows and/or pressures are required. Compressed air can be used for the delivery of aerosols, to power IPPB machines or mechanical ventilators, and to supply air to air/oxygen blenders, power tents, etc. This compressed gas can come from a main compressor, which is piped to rooms, or it can be generated by portable machines. Two of the main hazards associated with the use of portable machines are electrical safety and overheating of the compressor.

Laboratory Exercises

Obtain several air compressors of various sizes and perform the following exercises:

2-28. Using a manometer, check the maximum operating pressure of the compressor. Is it adjustable?

2-29. Using a flow measuring device, document the maximum flow rates obtainable from the compressor. Is there a relationship between flow rate and operating pressure?

2-30. Identify the alarms associated with the compressor.

Field Trips

2-31. *Local:* Locate the air compressor set-up providing the compressed air to your institution. Identify the system components.

2-32. *Extended:* Visit a manufacturer of air compressors.

REVIEW QUESTIONS

2-33. According to the United States Pharmacopeia, the purity of oxygen in cylinders must be at least:
A. 90.0%
B. 95.0%
C. 99.0%
D. 100%

2-34. Which of the following agencies makes recommendations governing the storage of gas cylinders?
A. NFPA
B. CGA
C. FDA
D. DOT

2-35. An E-cylinder contains 800 psig. How long will the cylinder last if 8 L/min is being used?
A. 6 min.
B. 16 min.
C. 26 min.
D. 36 min.

2-36. An H-cylinder with 1800 psig will last how long if 12 L/min is being used to drive a nebulizer at the 40% oxygen setting?
A. 3 hr, 23 min
B. 5 hr, 42 min
C. 7 hr, 51 min
D. 9 hr, 16 min

2-37. A cylinder filled with helium should be color coded:
A. green
B. brown
C. orange
D. gray

2-38. The oxygen safety system that functions to isolate sections on a hospital floor is called a:
A. station outlet
B. main shut-off valve
C. riser valve
D. zone valve

2-39. An E-cylinder of nitrous oxide is leaking gas. Which of the following would be appropriate actions?
I. replace the washer between the regulator and the tank
II. knock the pins off the regulator for a better fit
III. tighten the connections
IV. lubricate the leaking connection
A. I and II only
B. I and III only
C. I, III, and IV only
D. II, III, and IV only

2-40. Which of the following is most important for evaluating a home oxygen concentrator?
A.   sewer connections
B.   water system
C.   electrical load capacity
D.   number of rooms in the house

2-41. "Cracking" a cylinder prior to attachment of a regulator:
A.   demonstrates that there is some pressure in the cylinder
B.   helps remove "debris" from the valve outlet
C.   may result in cylinder damage
D.   all of the above
E.   A and B only

2-42. The American Standard Safety System is found on which of the following cylinders?
     I.   D
     II. E
     III. G
     IV. H
A.   I and II only
B.   III and IV only
C.   II, III, and IV only
D.   IV only

2-43. A pressure release valve on a cylinder would help prevent:
A.   excessive pressure from building up inside the cylinder
B.   tank rupture
C . inadvertent connection of an incorrect regulator attachment
D.   all of the above
E.   A and B only

2-44. Quick connect station outlets:
A.   help prevent incorrect gas delivery to a patient
B.   are part of the American Standard Safety System
C.   are closely regulated by strict governmental standards
D.   all of the above
E.   A and B only

2-45. To determine the contents of an E-cylinder of 100% CO_2, the practitioner must:
A.   only read the pressure gauge
B.   calculate contents by using the cylinder factor
C.   know the weight of the cylinder
D.   know the date when the cylinder was first in use

2-46. Use of an oxygen concentrator:
A.   will allow the delivery of 100% O_2 at all flow rates
B.   may require that a patient receive a higher flow rate of gas via a nasal cannula than they did while receiving cylinder oxygen
C.   always requires humidification since all models deliver a relative humidity of zero
D.   all of the above
E.   A and B only

2-47. Which of the following classifications would apply to gaseous oxygen?
      I.   flammable
      II. explosive
      III. supports combustion
      IV. nonflammable
  A.   I and II only
  B.   I and III only
  C.   II and III only
  D.   III and IV only

2-48. The most common method of oxygen production for commercial usage is:
  A.   electrolysis of water
  B.   heating of metallic oxides
  C.   peroxidation of water
  D.   the Joule-Kelvin method

2-49. Properties of helium which make it a valuable therapeutic gas include:
      I.   its low density
      II. ease of analysis
      III. chemical inertness
      IV. being nonflammable
  A.   I and III only
  B.   II and IV only
  C.   I, II, and III only
  D.   I, III, and IV only

2-50. Which of the following "gases" can be stored as a liquid at room temperature in a cylinder?
      I.   oxygen
      II. carbon dioxide
      III. helium
      IV. nitrous oxide
  A.   I and II only
  B.   I and III only
  C.   II and III only
  D.   II and IV only

3

Gas Delivery Systems: Regulators, Flowmeters, and Therapy Devices

INTRODUCTION

Oxygen is a drug, a fact that is often overlooked because of its routine use. The delivery of medical gases to patients, especially oxygen, is accomplished through the use of various types of respiratory therapy equipment. This chapter discusses the use of pressure reducing devices (regulators), flow controlling devices (flowmeters), and oxygen therapy devices which are responsible for providing an oxygen enriched environment.

SAFETY SYSTEMS

Chapter 2 describes two safety systems associated with tanks and regulators. The American Standard Safety System (ASSS), formerly known as the thread index safety system (TISS), and the Pin Index Safety System (PISS). ASSS connectors allow joining of a regulator with a large cylinder. PISS connectors allow joining of a regulator with a small cylinder. Another safety system, the Diameter Index Safety System (DISS), is also a threaded system similar to the ASSS, but it is used where pressures are less than 200 psig (connectors distal to the reducing valve). This adapter allows connection between flowmeters and other RT equipment. Two of the most commonly used type of connectors are for air and oxygen, each having a separate DISS designation. Although flowmeters are available with appropriate DISS adapters, many air flowmeters are manufactured with an oxygen DISS adapter. This allows interchanging of equipment among flowmeters and saves time, money, and equipment storage space. However, the availability of these adapters increases the chance of delivering an incorrect gas. Extra care must be taken to make sure the appropriate gas is being used. It is also important to note that not all threaded connectors are part of the safety systems described. The "permanent" connectors are pipe threads. They are not routinely unthreaded from their connectors.

REGULATORS

The typical regulator encountered in routine use is found connected to a gas cylinder. Regulators have three basic components, which perform three functions. Regulators have a pressure reducing valve or chamber for reducing pressures to an appropriate level. They have gauges for measuring cylinder contents. They also have a flow regulating/measuring device for controlling the flow of gas to be used. As stated in *Respiratory Care Equipment*, regulators may be classified as direct-acting or indirect-acting, single-stage or multistage, and as adjustable or nonadjustable (preset). The terms "adjustable" and "preset" refer to the method of operation of the device. Adjustable regulators allow change of flow to occur through the adjustment of pressure. Preset regulators are routinely set for a 50-psig outlet pressure, and flow is adjusted by means of a flow regulating device (Thorpe tube). These preset regulators can have their pressure adjusted by persons with the proper knowledge. They need to be checked for proper operation periodically and adjusted as needed to maintain outlet pressure at 50 psig.

Because most regulators are found attached to cylinders, it is important to understand the proper method to attach and remove them. Prior to attaching a regulator, the cylinder should be "cracked." This means the cylinder valve should opened and some gas allowed to escape. Cracking removes any dirt or debris in the cylinder outlet port and also demonstrates that the cylinder is pressurized.

Regulators with ASSS connectors can be threaded directly onto the cylinder. A large wrench is needed to tighten the adapter. Regulators with PISS adapters need a small plastic O-ring to create a seal between the regulator and the cylinder valve outlet so there is no leak. The yoke may be tightened by hand or with a small tool. Once the regulator is firmly in place, the tank valve should be pressurized. If a leak is heard, close the tank valve and recheck connectors. Before removing a regulator, the needle valve on the tank must be closed and the regulator depressurized.

FLOWMETERS

Devices that regulate and measure flow are commonly referred to as flowmeters. Flowmeters operate on the principle of a fixed or variable orifice. They are powered by a fixed or variable pressure. This results in a fixed or variable flow.

FLOW RESTRICTORS

Flow restrictors work off of a fixed pressure, have a fixed orifice, and deliver a fixed flow rate. Flow rate will decrease in the face of back-pressure.

BOURDON GAUGES

Bourdon gauges work off of a variable pressure, have a fixed orifice, and can deliver a variable flow rate. Bourdon gauges measure pressure. Those used to measure tank contents are calibrated in pressure units. Those used to indicate flow are calibrated in flow units. *Respiratory Care Equipment* describes the problems associated with the use of a pressure gauge to indicate flow. Bourdon gauges used to indicate flow will deliver less gas than indicated in the face of back-pressure.

An interesting note, though usually not clinically important, is that Bourdon gauges are aneroid pressure manometers. That is, they compare internal pressure to external pressure. If the gauge is exposed to an environment of increased atmospheric pressure (P_{atm}), it will record a lower reading even if the tank pressure remains the same. If exposed to a lower P_{atm}, the gauge will read higher.

THORPE TUBES

Thorpe tubes work off a fixed pressure, have a variable orifice, and can deliver a variable flow rate. Thorpe tubes can be divided into two general categories, back-pressure compensated and non–back-pressure compensated. Actual flow will be higher than indicated flow in the face of back-pressure with non–back-pressure-compensated Thorpe tubes. Consequently, they should not be used in clinical practice.

There are four methods to differentiate a back-pressure-compensated Thorpe tube from a non–back-pressure-compensated Thorpe tube.

1. Read the label on the flowmeter.
2. With the needle valve closed, plug the flowmeter into a pressurized gas source. The flow indicator (ball) will jump if it is a compensated flowmeter; it will not jump if the tube is uncompensated.
3. Measure the actual flow while applying back-pressure. Although both types of flowmeters will indicate decreased flow in the face of back-pressure, only the compensated tube will read accurately.
4. Dismantle the flowmeter and determine the placement of the needle valve. (Check text for further explanation.)

Thorpe tubes are calibrated to deliver accurate flow when operating at 760 mm Hg (1 P_{atm}), 70°F, and 50 psig internal pressure. Because of this, Thorpe tubes should never be used in combination with an adjustable regulator. Flowmeters are also calibrated for the density of the gas for which they are to be used. Inaccurate flows will result if gases of different densities from those for which the flowmeter is intended are delivered through a flowmeter of any type. Decreased density will result in increased flows; increased density will result in decreased flows.

Although Thorpe tubes must be upright to read the flow accurately, once the flow is set, placing a Thorpe tube on its side will not result in a change of flow. The needle valve controls the flow, not the ball. The ball only indicates the flow.

Thorpe tubes may come calibrated for different levels of flow: 0–1 L/min, 0–3 L/min, 0–15 L/min, or 0–75 L/min. Although they are calibrated for accurate flow, flows greater than the calibrated scale are possible as long as the outlet flow does not encounter excessive back-pressure. Many Thorpe type flowmeters set in the "flush" region will allow over 100 L/min unrestricted flow to exit from them when the needle valve is opened fully.

Laboratory Exercises

3-1. Compare the pressure release valve (pop-off) on a regulator to that on a gas cylinder.

3-2. Obtain both a pressure preset and pressure adjustable regulator. Compare the two regulators.

3-3. Disassemble and correctly reassemble a regulator identifying the following: gas inlet, gas outlet, pressure chamber, ambient chamber, diaphragm, spring, pressure gauge, and pressure release. Is it a direct-acting or indirect-acting pressure regulator?

3-4. Obtain the following flow measuring/regulating devices: Bourdon gauge, Thorpe tube, and flow restrictor. Compare them, classifying each as a fixed orifice/variable orifice, fixed pressure/variable pressure, and fixed flow/variable flow device.

3-5. Attach an adjustable regulator with a Bourdon gauge to a gas cylinder. Set the flow at 6 L/min. Completely occlude the outlet and observe the flow indicator.

3-6. Test a Thorpe tube flowmeter for back-pressure compensation by:
    1. Reading the label.
    2. With the needle valve closed, plugging it into a 50-psig gas source.
    3. Measuring the flow in the face of back-pressure.
    4. Determining the placement of the needle valve.

3-7. Obtain both back-pressure- and non–back-pressure-compensated Thorpe tubes. Connect them to a 50-psig gas source. Set the flow at 10 L/min and measure it. If it is accurate it should be delivering 10 L/min. Apply back-pressure to the flowmeters. What happens to the set flow compared to the actual flow with the pressure-compensated tube? The non–back-pressure-compensated tube?

3-8. Obtain a back-pressure-compensated Thorpe tube and connect it to an adjustable regulator. (*This should never be done in clinical practice!*) Using a pressure gauge, set the regulator at 20-psig outlet pressure. Adjust the flow on the flowmeter to 10 L/min. Measure the actual flow. How do they compare? Repeat this at 30, 40, 50, 60, 70, and 80 psig. Always reset the flow at 10 L/min before measuring the actual flow rate.

3-9. Attach a preset regulator with a Thorpe tube to an E-cylinder. Set the flow at 6 L/min and measure it. Now place the E-cylinder on its side and continue to measure the actual flow. What happens to the flow indicator? Does actual flow change?

3-10. Obtain a flow measuring device capable of measuring continuous flow at over 100 L/min. Place a Thorpe tube into a 50-psig wall outlet and slowly open the needle valve the whole way. Document the flow output.

OXYGEN THERAPY DEVICES

As described in *Respiratory Care Equipment,* oxygen therapy devices can be classified into two groups: low-flow, variable performance devices, or high-flow, fixed performance devices. The use of low-flow devices will result in a variable FIO_2 as the patient's respiratory rate, VT, I : E ratio, etc., change. In some cases, FIO_2 will vary with mouth or nose breathing. The use of high-flow devices will result in a constant FIO_2 regardless of the patient's breathing pattern. This is because high-flow devices are intended to meet or exceed the patient's inspiratory demand. High-flow devices include air-entrainment masks (AEMs), large-volume aerosol systems, large-volume humidifier systems, oxygen hoods, isolettes, and tents. Mechanical ventilators and IMV and CPAP systems would also fit into this category. Low-flow devices include nasal catheters, nasal cannulas, transtracheal catheters, simple masks, partial rebreathing masks (PRMs), and non-rebreathing masks (NRMs).

BRIEF SUMMARY OF DEVICES

The various types of oxygen therapy devices are explained in *Respiratory Care Equipment*. Following is a brief summary.

- **Nasal catheter**: Rarely used.
- **Nasal cannula**: Commonly used owing to ease of use and good tolerance by patients. Delivered FIO_2 is, however, difficult, if not impossible, to calculate or even estimate. It is the second best choice of the oxygen therapy devices for patients with COPD in acute exacerbations or in unstable conditions. Remember that cannulas are only useful if the patient has patent nasal passages.
- **Simple masks**: These devices should be last in line when considering the choices of oxygen therapy equipment. Low flows may result in rebreathing of CO_2 and heat build-up in the mask. If low FIO_2s are desired, an AEM should be used. If high FIO_2s are desired, a PRM or NRM should be used. A simple mask should be used when other oxygen equipment is unavailable. Some simple masks are manufactured with the small-bore oxygen tubing adapter made to entrain room air. This increases the total flow into the mask and helps maintain a more constant FIO_2.
- **Partial rebreathing and non-rebreathing masks**: These masks can deliver relatively high FIO_2s when using high flow rates and a tight-fitting mask. The premise that the first third of a patient's exhaled gas enters the reservoir bag when using a PRM needs further investigation. In some situations, the patient's exhaled gas will most likely take the path of least resistance, which is between a loosely fitting mask and the patient's face or through the exhalation valves with little gas entering the reservoir bag. The O_2 flow rate into the bag, the actual bag distention, and the patient's exhaled volume and flow rate also likely play a role in this matter.
- **Air-entrainment masks**: AEMs should be the oxygen delivery device of choice when a known FIO_2 is desired. They should be the first choice for patients with unstable COPD. After the acute exacerbation has passed, they may be exchanged for a cannula. For entrainment devices, the size of the jet and the size of the entrainment ports (windows) control the O_2 : air ratio and thus the FIO_2. Small jets result in increased room air entrainment and lower FIO_2s. Small ports allow less entrainment and increased FIO_2s. The source gas flow influences total gas flow but changes in source gas flow should not change the O_2 : air ratio and thus have minimal effects on the FIO_2.
- **Oxygen hoods**: These are used for treatment of neonates. They produce a controlled environment of temperature, humidity, and FIO_2. The flow of oxygen delivered by an oxygen hood should always be warmed and humidified. Temperature and FIO_2 should be constantly monitored. Suggested flows vary from a minimum of 7 L/min recommended for small hoods to 10–12 L/min minimum for large hoods. This flow should help guarantee that an appropriate FIO_2 will be maintained and that carbon dioxide will be washed out of the hood. Oxygen hoods can be used independently or in conjunction with an isolette.
- **Tents**: Tent therapy is most often used for older infants and pediatric patients. Goals of tent therapy include maintaining a constant FIO_2, maintaining a subambient temperature, delivery of humidity, and providing an isolated environment. Al-

though often referred to as "O_2 tents," compressed air can be used to power the tent if oxygen concentrations greater than 21% are not required. The FIO_2 in a tent will vary depending on the delivered FIO_2, the total flow into the tent, the tent canopy volume, how tightly the canopy fits the bed, and how often the canopy is opened and closed. Total flow into the tent (greater than 15 L/min) should be high enough to provide a constant FIO_2 and to wash out the CO_2 exhaled by the patient. The FIO_2s may vary from 0.21 to 0.50. Environmental temperature can be influenced by evaporative cooling (very inefficient), the use of ice, or the use of a refrigeration unit. This temperature will vary depending on the efficiency of the cooling unit, the size of the canopy, how well the canopy fits the bed, how often the canopy is opened, the room temperature, and possibly the patient's size and body temperature. Because a cool environment is usually desired during tent therapy, its use is not indicated for newborns, who require a warm environment. Humidity is delivered in the form of an aerosol via an atomizer or some type of nebulizer.

The term "croup tent" is also widely used because tents are a common method of treatment for patients with croup. Tents are also used for special purposes such as Ribavirin therapy for patients with bronchiolitis. Some of the hazards of tent therapy include: development of bronchospasms from the inhaled water particles, infection due to contaminated aerosols, difficulty of patient inspection in a dense aerosol, and a fire hazard with the increased oxygen environment. Electrical or spark-generating devices should not be allowed in or near a tent.

Laboratory Exercises

3-11. Obtain each of the following: a nasal cannula, an AEM, and an NRM. Appropriately place each of these devices on a manikin or classmate at the proper flow.

3-12. Obtain a 40% AEM. Set it up with the source gas flow at 10 L/min and analyze the FIO_2.
    1. Turn the source gas flow to 8 L/min and 12 L/min and reanalyze at each setting. What happens to the FIO_2?
    2. Block the entrainment ports and remeasure the FIO_2. What happens to the FIO_2?

REVIEW QUESTIONS

3-13. Line pressure in the hospital oxygen system should be approximately 50 psig because:
    A. it is a safe pressure
    B. most respiratory therapy equipment is manufactured to operate properly at 50 psig
    C. higher pressures would rupture gas lines
    D. all of the above

3-14. Two different manufacturers of AEMs have entrainment ports that are the same size, yet the delivered FIO_2 is different. This is due to:
    A. different jet sizes
    B. different mask designs
    C. different mask volumes
    D. different suggested source gas settings

3-15. A mist tent is producing less aerosol than it was earlier. Which of the following may be a source of the problem?

    I.   decreased air entrainment
    II. decreased coolant in the refrigeration unit
    III. partially obstructed nebulizer capillary tube
    IV. water level below the refill line

    A.   I and II only
    B.   I, II, and III only
    C.   I, III, and IV only
    D.   I, II, III, and IV

3-16. The reservoir bag of a non-rebreathing oxygen mask collapses during use. Appropriate action would be to:

    A.   remove the valves
    B.   replace the mask
    C.   increase the oxygen flow
    D.   tighten the mask on the patient's face

3-17. The approximate total flow delivered from a 50% AEM operating at 15 L/min is:

    A.   30 L/min
    B.   35 L/min
    C.   40 L/min
    D.   45 L/min

3-18. Which of the following are classified as high flow of fixed performance devices, delivering a constant FIO_2 regardless of ventilatory pattern?

    A.   AEMs
    B.   non-rebreathing masks
    C.   nasal cannulas
    D.   all of the above
    E.   A and B only

3-19. Room air will not enter the exhalation ports of an oxygen mask during inspiration if:

    A.   the mask is fitted tightly to the patient's face
    B.   total gas flow exceeds the patient's peak inspiratory flow rate
    C.   the source gas flow is set low
    D.   all of the above
    E.   A and B only

3-20. 40% oxygen is requested for a newborn infant. Which of the following is the best means for delivering the prescribed FIO_2?

    A.   cannula
    B.   simple mask
    C.   aerosol mask
    D.   oxygen hood

3-21. Which of the following will affect the FIO_2 delivered by a low-flow or variable oxygen delivery system?

    I.   respiratory rate
    II. equipment reservoir
    III. anatomic reservoir
    IV. patient's tidal volume

A. I and II only
B. I, III, and IV only
C. III and IV only
D. I, II, III, and IV

3-22. A patient has been on a nasal cannula at 2 L/min but exhibits a change in rate and depth of breathing. Which device would better meet the needs of this patient and maintain a constant FIO_2?
A. AEM at 28%
B. a simple mask at 8 L/min
C. a partial rebreathing mask at 12 L/min
D. a non-rebreathing mask at 15 L/min

3-23. A patient with COPD and elevated CO_2 levels presents to the Emergency Department with shortness of breath and cyanosis. The most appropriate oxygen administration device in this situation is a:
A. nasal cannula
B. AEM
C. simple mask
D. partial rebreathing mask

3-24. An AEM set at 28% with a source gas flow of 6 L/min will deliver a total flow of:
A. 72 L/min
B. 66 L/min
C. 60 L/min
D. 54 L/min

3-25. The accuracy of the Bourdon type flowmeters are affected by:
A. source pressure
B. position
C. downsteam resistance
D. flow rate delivered

3-26. A flowmeter allows continuous flow of gas with the needle valve completely closed. Which of the following is the most appropriate action?
A. check the wall outlet pressure
B. change the O-ring in the wall valve seat
C. replace the flowmeter
D. place a note on the flowmeter telling of the condition

4

Hyperbaric Oxygen Chambers and Related Respiratory Care Equipment

INTRODUCTION

Hyperbaric medicine deals with the process of delivering gases under pressure. Associated clinical applications and hazards are listed in *Respiratory Care Equipment*. During the application of hyperbaric medicine, the relationships of P, V, and T expressed in the gas laws (Chapter 1) are important considerations. Because the volume of the hyperbaric chamber is fixed, as P increases T will also increase. This is an application of Gay-Lussac's law. For this reason, it is important to flush the chamber with air during pressurization to maintain an appropriate temperature.

The application of Boyle's law is especially important during decompression. A loculated volume of gas will expand and gas bubbles will form in solution if decompression occurs too rapidly. If this phenomenon occurs in a patient's body, it can result in complications such as a pneumothorax, pulmonary gas emboli, tympanic membrane rupture, and sinus trauma.

Dalton's and Henry's laws are very important in a discussion dealing with hyperbaric oxygen therapy (HBO), since many of the benefits associated with HBO are due to the increased amount of O_2 that can be dissolved in the blood. To explain the benefit of hyperbaric medicine and its relationship to Dalton's and Henry's laws, the concepts of alveolar air equation and O_2 content will be discussed.

ALVEOLAR AIR EQUATION

Remember from Chapter 1 that $P_{atm} \times FIO_2 = PIO_2$ (the partial pressure of O_2 in the inspired gas under dry conditions). This formula must now be modified to include water vapor. For normal patient situations, water vapor pressure (PH_2O) is 47 mm Hg at 37°C and 100% relative humidity (refer to Chapter 5). The modified formula will now appear like this:

$$(P_{atm} - 47) \times FIO_2 = PIO_2$$

This calculation reduces the PIO_2 of air (dry) from 160 mm Hg ($760 \times .21 = 160$) to a PIO_2 of air (humidified) of 150 mm Hg ($[760 - 47] \times .21 = 150$)

The alveolar air equation takes the above formula one step further and allows the calculation of PAO_2 (the partial pressure of oxygen in the alveoli). It is based on the P_{atm}, FIO_2, $PaCO_2$, and the R factor and is expressed in the following formula:

$$PAO_2 = (P_{atm} - 47)(FIO_2) - PaCO_2 (FIO_2 + [(1 - FIO_2)/R])$$

It is often simplified to this form:

$$PAO_2 = (P_{atm} - 47)(FIO_2) - PaCO_2/R$$

where:

- PAO_2 is the alveolar PO_2 in mm Hg
- P_{atm} is atmospheric pressure or the barometric pressure (pressure measured by a barometer), expressed in mm Hg. In this case, it is also the absolute pressure to which the patient is exposed.
- 47 is the water vapor pressure (PH_2O) in mm Hg in a person's lungs at 37°C and 100% relative humidity (RH)
- FIO_2 is the fractional concentration of inhaled O_2
- $PaCO_2$ is the arterial CO_2 value in mm Hg
- R is the respiratory exchange ratio (RER), the actual mean ratio of CO_2/O_2 exchanged in the lung. *Note:* There are several factors that will affect the actual R value; their discussion is beyond the scope of this text. A value of 0.8 is considered normal and is commonly used in the formula unless the patients actual R value is known. When patients are breathing 100% O_2, R will be given a value of 1, thus eliminating it from the formula.

Examples

Example A
While breathing room air at 1 P_{atm} of 760 mm Hg, the PIO_2 is approximately 150 mm Hg. A person with a normal $PaCO_2$ of 40 mm Hg will have a PAO_2 of approximately 100 mm Hg.

$$PIO_2 = (760 - 47)(.21) - 40/.8$$

$$PIO_2 = 713 \times .21 - 50$$

$$PAO_2 = 150 - 50 = 100 \text{ mm Hg}$$

Example B

Breathing room air (21% O_2) under 2 P_{atm} results in the following values: PIO_2 of 309 and a PAO_2 of 259.

$$PIO_2 = (2 \times 760 - 47)(.21) - 40/.8$$

$$PAO_2 = 1473 \times .21 - 50$$

$$PAO_2 = 309 - 50 = 259 \text{ mm Hg}$$

Note that $PH2O$ does not change with changes in pressure (refer to Chapter 5) and that the situation is *equivalent* to breathing approximately 43% O_2 at 1 P_{atm}. [309/(760 – 47) = .43 or 43%].

Example C

Under 2 P_{atm}, while breathing 100% O_2, the PAO_2 will go much higher.

$$PAO_2 = (2 \times 760 - 47)(1.0) - 40$$

$$PAO_2 = 1473 \times 1 - 40$$

$$PAO_2 = 1473 - 40 = 1433 \text{ mm Hg}$$

This phenomenon directly affects the possibility of increased PaO_2 (partial pressure of O_2 in the arterial blood) since the amount of oxygen dissolved in the plasma is directly affected by the PAO_2.

PIO_2, PAO_2 Calculations: Student Exercise

Calculate the PIO_2 and PAO_2 for each of the following conditions. PH_2O will be 47 mm Hg for each of the calculations, and 1 P_{atm} (in Problems 4-7 and 4-8) will be equal to 760 mm Hg.

	P_{atm} (mm Hg)	FIO_2	$PaCO_2$ (mm Hg)	PIO_2 (mm Hg)	PAO_2 (mm Hg)
4-1.	760	.30	40	_____	_____
4-2.	760	1.0	40	_____	_____
4-3.	760	.21	60	_____	_____
4-4.	620	.21	40	_____	_____
4-5.	620	.50	20	_____	_____
4-6.	360	.21	20	_____	_____
4-7.	3 P_{atm}	.21	40	_____	_____
4-8.	3 P_{atm}	1.0	40	_____	_____

OXYGEN CONTENT

The O_2 content of blood (arterial, CaO_2, or venous, CvO_2) is determined by the amount of O_2 dissolved in the plasma and the amount of O_2 carried on the hemoglobin (Hb). It is commonly expressed by the following formula:

$$O_2 \text{ content} = (0.003 \times PO_2) + (Hb \times O_2 \text{ Sat} \times 1.34)$$

where:
- 0.003 is the solubility coefficient for O_2 in mL of O_2/dL of blood/mm Hg.
- PO_2 is the PO_2 in arterial blood (PaO_2) or the PO_2 in venous blood (PvO_2).
- Hb is the grams (g) of Hb present in 100 mL of blood (g/100 mL) (g%).
- O_2 Sat is the saturation of Hb with O_2 (expressed here as a fraction).
- 1.34 is a constant, representing the maximum amount (mL) of O_2 that can be carried by one g of Hb (mL / g Hb) when Hb is 100% filled or saturated with oxygen. *Note:* Although 1.36 and 1.39 have been used in some texts for O_2 content determination, 1.34 will be used for this discussion.

The O_2 content can be expressed in milliliters of O_2 per 100 mL of blood, or milliliters of O_2 per deciliter of blood, or as volumes %.

Examples

Example A
For a "normal" individual with a PaO_2 of 100 mm Hg, a Hb of 15 g, and a %Sat of 98%, the arterial O_2 content would be:

$$CaO_2 = (0.003 \times 100) + (15 \times .98 \times 1.34)$$

$$CaO_2 = .3 + 19.7 = 20.0 \text{ mL } O_2/\text{dL blood}$$

Example B
When breathing 100% O_2 at 1 P_{atm}, the PaO_2 can reach levels as high as 600 mm Hg. This has the potential of raising the CaO_2 somewhat, but content is limited since Hb is already 98% filled at a PaO_2 of 100 and the solubility coefficient is so low at 0.003.

$$CaO_2 = (0.003 \times 600) + (15 \times 1.0 \times 1.34)$$

$$CaO_2 = 1.8 + 20.1 = 21.9 \text{ mL } O_2/\text{dL blood}$$

Example C
Breathing 100% O_2 at 3 P_{atm} has the potential of increasing O_2 content much more:

$$CaO_2 = (0.003 \times 2000) + (15 \times 1.0 \times 1.34)$$

$$CaO_2 = 6 + 20.1 = 26.1 \text{ mL } O_2 / \text{dL blood}$$

At this level of PaO_2 it is possible for the plasma to supply all the O_2 needed. Oxygen on the hemoglobin need not be unloaded. In theory, a person would not need Hb for O_2 delivery at this level of PaO_2. One of the main purposes for using hyperbaric medicine for treatment of various conditions is to increase the O_2 dissolved in the plasma for ultimate delivery to cells.

Oxygen Content Calculations: Student Exercise

Calculate the CaO_2 for the following conditions:

	PaO_2 (mm Hg)	Hb (g%)	O_2 Sat	CaO_2 (mL O_2/dL blood)
4-9.	100	15	98	_____
4-10.	60	15	90	_____
4-11.	40	15	75	_____
4-12.	40	20	75	_____
4-13.	60	10	90	_____
4-14.	100	5	98	_____
4-15.	400	10	100	_____

DIVING AND HYPERBARICS

Divers are affected by the same principles of hyperbarics. Since divers do not require high PaO_2 levels, they can avoid some of the risks involved with hyperbaric medicine by breathing He/O_2 mixtures (with less than 21% O_2) for deep dives and for long submersion periods. Breathing He/O_2 mixtures decreases the chances of both pulmonary and systemic O_2 toxicity. The decreased density of a He/O_2 mixture also makes breathing easier (decreases resistance to flow) when compared to breathing room air. This is an application of Poiseuille's law for turbulent flow.

HYPOBARIC CONDITIONS

Although the objective of this chapter is to discuss HBO, it is important to mention hypobaric conditions (pressures less than one normal atmospheric pressure). Routinely, pressures less than 1 P_{atm} are acutely experienced when ascending to high altitudes during flight, or driving up a mountain such as Pikes Peak in Colorado. It is chronically experienced by those who live at high altitudes. Ascent to high altitudes results in decompression, and the principles and hazards described with decompression from hyperbaric conditions apply. However, the magnitude is usually less. Both acute ascents and high-altitude dwelling result in PIO_2 and PaO_2 values lower than the "normal" values due to the atmospheric pressure being less than the 760 mm Hg at sea level. If blood oxygen levels drop significantly, hypoxemia can result. This can cause hyperventilation and acute altitude sickness which is often manifested by headache, fatigue, dizziness, nausea, loss of appetite, and palpitations.

PO_2 Calculations: Student Exercise

Calculate the following. Assume a normal $PaCO_2$ and a P_{atm} equal to 760 mm Hg unless stated otherwise.

4-16. Calculate the PIO_2 and PAO_2 if room air is inspired under hyperbaric conditions of 1.5 P_{atm}.

4-17. Calculate the PIO_2 and PAO_2 if 100% O_2 is inspired under hyperbaric conditions of 2.5 P_{atm}.

4-18. Calculate the PIO_2 and PO_2 if 21% O_2 is inspired at 0.5 P_{atm}.

4-19. Calculate the PIO_2 and PAO_2 if 40% O_2 is inspired at 0.5 P_{atm}.

Clinical Problem Solving: Student Exercise

4-20. If a hyperbaric chamber could be instantaneously pressurized to 2 P_{atm}, what would the resultant temperature be in degrees Fahrenheit if the initial temperature was 72°F?

4-21. A patient is receiving hyperbaric therapy at 2.5 P_{atm}. A lung segment, after stabilizing at 500 mL, develops complete bronchial obstruction. If the chamber rapidly depressurizes to 1.5 P_{atm}, what will happen to the volume of the lung segment? Calculate the change.

4-22. According to Avagadro's law, the density of a gas is expressed as the gram molecular weight (gmw) of the gas divided by 22.4 L. For O_2 it is 32/22.4 or 1.43 g/L. If 1 gmw of O_2 is compressed to 11.2 L, what will be the density of O_2?

4-23. According to Poiseuille's law for turbulent flow, what happens to air flow resistance as gas density increases? What will happen to the work of breathing?

4-24. Calculate the amount of O_2 bound to hemoglobin, and that dissolved in the plasma when under 2 P_{atm} of pressure with 100% O_2. O_2 Sat = 100%, Hb = 13, and PaO_2 = 1100 mm Hg.

REVIEW QUESTIONS

4-25. Which of the following would be considered hazards of hyperbaric chambers?
    A.   chamber fires
    B.   decompression pneumothorax
    C.   pulmonary gas emboli
    D.   all of the above
    E.   A and B only

4-26. The psig associated with 3 P_{atm} is:
    A.   0 psig
    B.   14.7 psig
    C.   29.4 psig
    D.   44.1 psig

4-27. Although some ventilators have demonstrated minimal effects when exposed to high environmental pressures (i.e., hyperbaric chambers), in general which of the following are correct?
    A.   tidal volume delivery decreases
    B.   minute ventilation decreases
    C.   machine frequency increases
    D.   all of the above
    E.   A and B only

4-28. Relative contraindications of HBO include:
    A.   pneumothorax
    B.   obstructive bronchial disease
    C.   confinement anxiety

  D. all of the above

  E. A and B only

4-29. Complications associated with HBO when breathing high oxygen concentrations may include:

  A. pulmonary oxygen toxicity

  B. systemic oxygen toxicity

  C. increased airway flow resistance

  D. all of the above

  E. A and B only

4-30. To help reduce the hazards of hyperbarics, divers should breathe, along with some oxygen:

  A. a high N_2 concentration

  B. a high CO_2 concentration

  C. a high He concentration

  D. a high CO concentration

4-31. The solubility coefficient for oxygen is:

  A. 3.0 mL of O_2/dL of blood/mm Hg

  B. 0.3 mL of O_2/dL of blood/mm Hg

  C. 0.03 mL of O_2/dL of blood/mm Hg

  D. 0.003 mL of O_2/dL of blood/mm Hg

4-32. A patient in an HBO chamber is breathing compressed air at an absolute pressure of 1900 mm Hg. This would be equivalent to breathing what concentration of oxygen at 1 P_{atm} (760 mm Hg)?

  A. 28%

  B. 35%

  C. 53%

  D. 74%

  E. 86%

5

Humidification: Humidifiers and Nebulizers

INTRODUCTION

Chapter 5 deals mainly with humidification of gases and the equipment used to achieve it. The following exercises will allow a review of the concepts involved with gas humidification.

WATER VAPOR PRESSURE

Like other gases, molecular water in the environment (water vapor) exerts a partial pressure, water vapor pressure (PH_2O). At 37°C and 100% relative humidity (RH), each liter of gas holds 43.9 mg of H_2O (0.0439 mL) and exerts a partial pressure of 47 mm Hg. Unlike other gases, PH_2O is not dependent on the total pressure in a system but on the amount of actual water present in a gas sample.

Examples

Use Table 5-1 in *Respiratory Care Equipment* to confirm these values.

Example A
A dry gas sample at 0% RH, 37°C, and 760 mm Hg contains 0 mg of H_2O and has a PH_2O of 0 mm Hg.

Example B
A gas sample at 100% RH, 20°C and 760 mm Hg contains 17.3 mg of H_2O/L and has a PH_2O of 17.5 mm Hg.

Example C
A gas sample at 100% RH, 37°C and 760 mm Hg contains 43.9 mg of H_2O/L and has a PH_2O of 47 mm Hg.

41

Example D

A gas sample at 100% RH, 37°C, and 560 mm Hg contains 43.9 mg of H_2O/L and has a PH_2O of 47 mm Hg.

Example E

A gas sample at 100% RH, 37°C, and 2 P_{atm} contains 43.9 mg of H_2O/L and has a PH_2O of 47 mm Hg.

Example F

A gas sample at 50% RH, 37°C, and 760 mm Hg contains approximately 22 mg of H_2O/L and has a PH_2O of approximately 22 mm Hg.

Although total system pressure affects the partial pressure of other gases in the system, it does not affect PH_2O. Another important point is that PH_2O must be accounted for before calculating the partial pressure of any other gas in the system. That is why PH_2O is always subtracted from the P_{atm} prior to multiplying by the FIO_2 in the alveolar air equation. (Refer to Chapter 4.) Water vapor pressure PH_2O always takes its "piece of the pie" first.

Absolute Humidity and PH_2O Calculations: Student Exercise

Calculate the absolute humidity and the PH_2O under each of the following conditions. Use Table 5-1 in *Respiratory Care Equipment* to determine the values.

	Temperature	RH	Absolute Humidity (mg/L)	PH_2O (mm Hg)
5-1.	37°C	50%	_____	_____
5-2.	40°C	100%	_____	_____
5-3.	24°C	100%	_____	_____
5-4.	24°C	25%	_____	_____
5-5.	30°C	75%	_____	_____

Humidified P_{gas} Calculations: Student Exercise

Calculate the PO_2 and PN_2 for each of the following gas mixtures of O_2, N_2, and H_2O. Use the answers from the previous problems for determining the PH_2O to be used here.

	%O_2	Pres (mm Hg)	Temp (°C)	%RH	PO_2 (mm Hg)	PN_2 (mm Hg)
5-6.	21	760	37	0	_____	_____
5-7.	21	760	37	50	_____	_____
5-8.	21	760	40	100	_____	_____
5-9.	40	620	24	100	_____	_____
5-10.	40	620	24	25	_____	_____
5-11.	21	760	30	75	_____	_____

STPD, ATPS, AND BTPS

STPD, ATPS, and BTPS are conditions of varied pressure, temperature, and humidification. The volume of a gas will change when it is converted from one set of conditions to another.

STPD is Standard Temperature, Pressure, Dry
  Standard temperature is 0°C.
  Standard pressure is one atmospheric pressure at 760 mm Hg.
  Dry means there is no water vapor.

ATPS is Ambient Temperature, Pressure, Saturated with water
  Ambient temperature is the actual temperature in the given situation.
  Ambient pressure is the actual atmospheric pressure.
  Saturated means that the gas at the ambient temperature is carrying all of the water it can. (RH=100%)

BTPS is Body Temperature, Pressure, Saturated with water
  Body temperature is 37°C.
  Body pressure is ambient pressure.
  Saturated means that the gas at 37°C is carrying all the water that it can. (RH=100%)

Note: Pulmonary function values are *all* routinely corrected to BTPS except the DLCO which is reported at STPD. Other values such as O_2 consumption and CO_2 production are also routinely reported at STPD.

MANUAL CONVERSION BETWEEN STPD, ATPS, AND BTPS

Manual conversions between the conditions (STPD, ATPS, and BTPS) can be done by two basic methods. These include conversion factors from tables and the use of the combined gas law. The use of the conversion factors is the most common.

Examples

Example of Method 1

What lung volume will result on inhalation of 4 L of air at 24°C, 760 mm Hg and saturated with water vapor? (ATPS to BTPS conversion)

To solve, go to the correct conversion tables (for this conversion use Table 5-1), find the appropriate factor, and, in this case, multiply the factor times the initial volume.

$$4 \text{ L (ATPS)} \times 1.08 = 4.32 \text{ L (BTPS)}$$

Note that 4 L of gas inhaled at room temperature will "expand" to 4.32 L in the lungs. This is a result of two factors: warming of the gas, and addition of water vapor or humidification of the gas. If the reverse, a BTPS to ATPS conversion, is desired, the factor would be divided into the volume instead of multiplying.

$$4.32 \text{ L (BTPS)}/1.08 = 4.0 \text{ L (ATPS)}$$

TABLE 5-1. ATPS to BTPS Volume Conversion Factors for Common Ambient Temperatures at or Near 760 mm Hg Pressure	
Temperature (°C)	BTPS Factor
20	1.102
21	1.096
22	1.091
23	1.085
24	1.080
25	1.075
26	1.068

Example of Method 2

This method utilizes the combined gas law for the conversion. This time water vapor must be considered when using the combined gas law, which was not taken into account in Chapter 1.

Using the same values as in the first example employing Method 1, the conversion would look like this (ATPS to BTPS):

$$\frac{P_1V_1}{T_1} = \frac{P_2V_2}{T_2} \qquad \frac{(760-22)4}{297} = \frac{(760-47)V_2}{310} \qquad V_2 = 4.32$$

In this example using Method 2, 22 is the P_{H_2O} at 24°C, and 47 is the P_{H_2O} at 37°C. Both are at 100% RH.

Remember that the temperatures must be expressed as absolute temperature values. Although it is more time consuming, Method 2 allows conversions from any set of conditions to any other set of conditions, whereas the charts limit the choices.

STPD, ATPS, BTPS Calculations: Student Exercise

Calculate each of the following (try comparing Method 1 to Method 2). Use Tables 5-1, 5-2, and 5-3 to aid in the calculations.

5-12.   1 L STPD to BTPS (BP = 750)   _____

5-13.   3 L STPD to ATPS (BP = 740, T = 20°C)   _____

5-14.   5 L BTPS (BP = 770) to STPD   _____

5-15.   2 L BTPS (BP = 760) to ATPS (BP = 760, T = 25°C)   _____

5-16.   6 L ATPS (BP = 760, T = 22°C) to BTPS (BP = 760)   _____

5-17.   4 L ATPS (BP = 756, T = 26°C) to STPD   _____

5-18.   6 L ATPD (BP = 660, T = 24°C) to BTPS (BP = 660)   _____
        (D = dry):   *Use Method 2 **only** for 5-18*

TABLE 5-2. STPD to BTPS Volume Conversion Factors at Various Barometric Pressures

Pressure (mm Hg)	Factor
740	1.245
742	1.241
744	1.238
746	1.235
748	1.232
750	1.227
752	1.224
754	1.221
756	1.217
758	1.214
760	1.211
762	1.208
764	1.203
766	1.200
768	1.196
770	1.193

TABLE 5-3. ATPS to STPD Volume Conversion Factors at Various Temperatures and Pressures

P_{atm}	20°C	21°C	22°C	23°C	24°C	25°C	26°C
740	0.883	0.878	0.874	0.869	0.864	0.860	0.855
742	0.885	0.881	0.876	0.871	0.867	0.862	0.857
744	0.888	0.883	0.878	0.874	0.869	0.864	0.859
746	0.890	0.886	0.881	0.876	0.872	0.867	0.862
748	0.892	0.888	0.883	0.879	0.874	0.869	0.864
750	0.895	0.890	0.886	0.881	0.876	0.872	0.867
752	0.897	0.893	0.888	0.883	0.879	0.874	0.869
754	0.900	0.895	0.891	0.886	0.881	0.876	0.872
756	0.902	0.898	0.893	0.888	0.883	0.879	0.874
758	0.905	0.900	0.886	0.891	0.886	0.881	0.876
760	0.907	0.902	0.898	0.893	0.888	0.883	0.879
762	0.910	0.905	0.900	0.896	0.891	0.886	0.881
764	0.912	0.907	0.903	0.898	0.893	0.888	0.884
766	0.915	0.910	0.905	0.900	0.896	0.891	0.886
768	0.917	0.912	0.908	0.903	0.898	0.893	0.888
770	0.919	0.915	0.910	0.905	0.901	0.896	0.891

HUMIDIFIERS

Because the amount of H_2O vapor a gas can contain is based primarily on its temperature, unheated humidifiers regardless of their construction or type are very inefficient.

Example

Water is placed in a bubble humidifier and O_2, at 6 L/min, is bubbled through the water. Due to evaporation of the water, the temperature of the water begins to drop. Assume the temperature of the water and the gas passing through it decreases to 16°C and the humidifier is able to deliver 100% RH under those conditions. The actual amount of H_2O in the gas would be 13.6 mg/L. The amount of humidity delivered by a device is often converted to %RH at body conditions. When converted to % RH at body temperature, the RH of the gas leaving the humidifier would be 13.6/43.9 or 31%.

Laboratory Exercises

5-19. Obtain several humidifiers and compare their construction and method of operation.

5-20. Fill a bubble humidifier with water. Allow it to stand for a period of time so the temperature can equilibrate with room temperature. Document the temperature of the water. Bubble O_2 through the humidifier at various flow rates (2, 4, 6, 8 L/min) for a period of time, allowing the temperature to stabilize at each of the flow settings. Document the temperatures. What happens to the water temperature as flow rates increase? Why? How will this affect humidity output at different flow rates?

5-21. Fill a bubble humidifier with water and weigh it. A very accurate weight is needed. Bubble O_2 through the humidifier at a set flow rate for a set period of time. Consider at least 24 hours. At the end of the period of time, measure the temperature of the water and weigh the humidifier and the remaining water again. The difference in the weight is the H_2O evaporated during the time period. Divide the milligrams of water evaporated by the total number of liters of gas that passed through the humidifier. The result will be the mean water content of each liter of gas. From this, the RH of the delivered gas can be calculated at the actual temperature and at BTPS. Repeat this exercise at different flow rates and with various types of humidifiers.

5-22. Routinely the pressure release or "pop-off" of a bubble humidifier is set at 2 psi. Document the pressure release value with a manometer by measuring the pressure inside the humidifier while causing activation of the pressure release.

Research Project

Manufacturers are constantly producing new humidifiers and new designs. Test the water output of these devices and report the RH produced.

HUMIDITY DEFICIT

Humidity deficit (HD) is the difference between the actual amount of water delivered per liter of gas and that which is needed at body temperature to make up 100% RH in the airway at 37°C. If the amount of humidity delivered is less than 43.9 mg/L, the water deficit must be added by the airways to the incoming gas. In the previous example with the bubble humidifier, only 13.6 mg of water were delivered per liter of gas passing through it. Considering only this flow of gas, the humidity deficit would be 43.9 – 13.6 or 30.3 mg/L. Increased humidity deficits will tend to dry secretions in the airways leading to other pulmonary complications. Note that during clinical use, low-flow humidifiers are responsible for humidifying only a part of the patient's inhaled gases. Much of the patient's inhaled gas may be room air. For actual calculation of humidity deficit of all of the inhaled gas, the conditions of the room air and the proportion of O_2 to room air inhaled would need to be known. Because bubble humidifiers are relatively inefficient and often provide humidification to only a fraction of the inhaled gas, their routine use has been discontinued by many Respiratory Care departments.

Humidity Deficit Calculations: Student Exercise

Calculate the humidity deficit for each of the following conditions:

5-23. O_2 flowing at 2 L/min via nasal cannula with the bubble humidifier water temperature at 20°C and 100% RH.

5-24. O_2 flowing at 6 L/min via simple mask with the bubble humidifier water temperature at 18°C and 80% RH.

5-25. O_2 flowing, unhumidified, at 12 L/min into a non-rebreathing mask.

NEBULIZERS

Nebulizers are aerosol generators that produce particles of water. Aerosol output is the total milligrams of water leaving the nebulizer per time period. Aerosol density is the milligrams of water per liter of gas produced by the nebulizer. Aerosol output and density will vary as total flow from a nebulizer changes. Although the purpose of aerosols is for "wetting down" the airway, some nebulizers only wet the patient's face and deliver a "dry" aerosol. That is, their density is less than 43.9 mg/L. Thus, a HD may still be present. This situation is more likely to occur with the use of jet nebulizers than it would with the use of the Babington or ultrasonic nebulizers (USN).

Laboratory Exercise

5-26. Obtain several types of nebulizers and compare their construction and method of operation.

5-27. Fill a jet nebulizer with H_2O and weigh it. A very accurate weight is needed. Power the nebulizer at a 40% entrainment setting with a predetermined flow rate from an O_2 flow meter for a set time period. (Consider 4–6 hours.) At the end of the time period, weigh the nebulizer and remaining H_2O again. The difference in weight is the amount of H_2O nebulized (and evaporated) by the nebulizer. Calculate the total flow for the given time period during which the nebulizer was in operation. Divide the mg of H_2O nebulized by the total flow output in liters. The result will be the milligrams of water per liter of gas flow. Was the density of the aerosol high enough to meet the airway needs at BTPS? (A graduated cylinder could be used to measure the amount of H_2O at the beginning and end, but it will not be as accurate as weighing it.) Repeat this exercise at different flow and entrainment settings and for the Babington and USN. If a better estimate of the aerosol density that actually reaches the patient is desired, include a 6-ft length of widebore tubing as part of the system. Include it in the initial and final weight without draining any of the water that collects in the tubing.

Research Project

Manufacturers are constantly producing new and updated models and designs of nebulizers. Measure the aerosol output of these devices and report the results.

TOTAL FLOW OUTPUT

When working with nebulizers and other entrainment devices, another important consideration is the total flow output of the device. Entrainment devices are classified as high-flow systems and should therefore provide enough flow output to meet the inspiratory flow rates of the patient. The purpose for meeting the patient's inspiratory demands is to make sure that the patient is receiving the appropriate FIO_2 as delivered by the device. If the flow rate delivered from the device is too low, the patient will inhale room air along with the FIO_2 delivered by the device, thus diluting the delivered FIO_2.

Routinely patients receiving O_2 from a high-flow system do not have their inspiratory flow rate (FR), inspiratory time (T_i) or tidal volume (V_t) measured. If resting peak inspiratory flow rate was known, the output from the system could be set to match it. If T_i and V_t were known, the average inspiratory flow rate could be calculated by the following formula:

$$FR \text{ (L/min)} = V_t \text{ (L)} \times 60 \text{ (sec/min)} / T_i \text{ (sec)}$$

Knowing these parameters would help guide the use of appropriate flow output from the entrainment device. Since FR, T_i, and V_t are not usually known, practitioners guess at the appropriate flow rates. A flow of 30 to 40 L/min would be a recommended minimum for these devices when used with adults. For many patients a flow of 60 L/min or greater would be more appropriate. If an aerosol is being delivered, the necessary flow rate can be estimated by observing the patient during inspiration. If the aerosol exiting the mask or T-piece "disappears" from the exhalation port during inspiration, the flow from the device may need to be increased.

Calculation of Total Flow Output

The total flow rate (FR_t) delivered from an entrainment device can be calculated by knowing the source gas flow rate (FR_{sg}, the O_2 flow meter setting) and the ratio of air to oxygen for the delivered FIO_2. (Refer to Chapter 1.) For a given FIO_2, add the ratio value for air (A) to the ratio value for O_2 (which is always 1) and then multiply that value by the flowmeter setting. This relationship is expressed in the following formula:

$$FR_t = FR_{sg}(A + O_2 \text{ ratio values})$$

Example

41% O_2 is being delivered with a flowmeter set at 8 L/min. What is the total flow being delivered to the patient? The A : O_2 ratio is 3 : 1.

$$FR_t = 8\,(3 + 1) = 8 \times 4 = 32\ \text{L/min}$$

Total Flow Calculations: Student Exercise

Calculate the total flow from entrainment devices under the following conditions:

	FIO$_2$ Setting (%)	Flow Setting (L/min)	Total Flow (L/min)
5-28.	41	12	_____
5-29.	37	10	_____
5-30.	34	10	_____
5-31.	28	6	_____
5-32.	24	3	_____
5-33.	47	12	_____
5-34.	60	15	_____
5-35.	70	15	_____

Critical Thinking Exercises

5-36. Why do many nebulizers, set at 55–60% or higher, need to be paired with a second nebulizer to deliver appropriate flow of gas?

5-37. What happens to a nebulizer's operation as water accumulates in the wide-bore tubing creating back pressure?

5-38. A physician orders a 40% O_2 aerosol mask via ultrasonic nebulizer. How can this be achieved?

5-39. A nebulizer, set at 8 L/min and 40% O_2, is analyzed at 40% O_2. If the source flow is now increased to 12 L/min, what will happen to the FIO_2?

5-40. A heated humidifier is being used to deliver humidity to a patient intubated with an endotracheal tube. The tubing between the patient and the humidifier constantly fills with water.
   a. Why is this happening?
   b. If the patient is receiving 50% oxygen via blender and flowmeter, will the water collecting in the tubing have an effect on the FIO_2?

For each of the following situations, diagnose the problem and state the appropriate action to be taken.

5-41. A respiratory care practitioner (RCP) is walking past the room of a patient who is receiving humidified O_2 via nasal cannula. Coming from the room is a popping noise or whistle. What is the noise and why is it occurring?

5-42. A patient is receiving O_2 at 4 L/min via nasal cannula. The patient comments to the RCP that he does not feel any flow coming from the cannula. The flow is set at 4 L/min, there are bubbles in the humidifier, and the tubing is connected.

5-43. A jet nebulizer with wide-bore tubing, a Briggs' adapter (T-piece), and a tail is set up and analyzed at 40% O_2. Later, while using another analyzer to recheck the FIO_2, it reads 60%. The analyzer is working properly and the entrainment port was not changed. Use this scenario for the following situations.

Situation 1. The practitioner hears a bubbling noise coming from the system.

Situation 2. The practitioner observes the end of the wide bore tubing pressed against the patients mattress after the patient was repositioned.

Situation 3. Due to lack of supplies, the practitioner had to find adapters with a very small diameter T-connector to measure the in-line FIO_2.

METERED DOSE INHALERS

Metered dose inhalers (MDIs) are aerosol generators used for medication delivery but not for humidification. There are many types of MDIs currently on the market. Regardless of the type of inhaler, as they are used they become empty and need to be replaced. Relative fullness can be determined simply by dropping the canister into a water bath. A full inhaler will sink, a partially filled inhaler will float upright, and one that is empty or almost so will float on its side.

REVIEW QUESTIONS

5-44. When using an air-entrainment device, and resistance to flow occurs downstream from the device, which of the following are true?

    I.   total flow decreases

    II.   total flow increases

    III.   the FIO_2 decreases

    IV.   the FIO_2 increases

  A.   I and III

  B.   I and IV

  C.   II and III

  D.   II and IV

5-45. The ability of humidifiers to humidify gas depends on which of the following factors?
A.   time of contact
B.   temperature of the system
C.   surface area of contact
D.   all of the above
E.   A and B only

5-46. Calculate the humidity deficit of a patient with a normal body temperature while breathing gas that is 57% humidified at body temperature.
A.   26.7 mg/L
B.   25 mg/L
C.   20.2 mg/L
D.   18.9 mg/L
E.   16.2 mg/L

5-47. Given a large-volume nebulizer set at 37% FIO_2 and driven by an oxygen flow rate of 12 L/min, calculate the total flow to the patient.
A.   30 L/min
B.   45 L/min
C.   60 L/min
D.   75 L/min

5-48 The approximate amount of water present in normal alveolar gas is:
A.   38 mg/L
B.   40 mg/L
C.   42 mg/L
D.   44 mg/L
E.   47 mg/L

5-49. Which of the following incorporates the use of a piezoelectric transducer?
A.   cascade humidifier
B.   ultrasonic nebulizer
C.   spinning disk nebulizer
D.   a SPAG unit

5-50. An intubated patient is receiving 50% oxygen from a jet nebulizer via T-piece (Briggs') adapter. Each time the patient inhales, the mist disappears. Appropriate action would include which of the following?
   I.   add a reservoir to the T-piece
   II. increase the flowmeter setting
   III. increase the FIO_2 setting on the nebulizer
A.   I only
B.   I and II
C.   II and III
D.   I, II, and III

5-51. Compared to unheated humidifiers, a major advantage of the heated humidifiers is that:
A.   particles are produced in the therapeutic range
B.   both molecular and particulate water are produced
C.   a baffle is not needed
D.   100% RH is easily attained at body temperature

5-52. Factors affecting the concentration of oxygen delivered by an entrainment device include:

      I.   the flow rate of oxygen powering the device

      II. size of the entrainment ports

      III. downstream obstruction

  A.   I only

  B.   I and II

  C.   II and III

  D.   I, II, and III

5-53. Which of the following would have the greatest humidity output potential?

  A.   a USN

  B.   a bubble humidifier

  C.   a jet nebulizer

  D.   a passover humidifier

5-54. The calculated humidity deficit while breathing room air at 20°C with a RH of 25% is approximately:

  A.   40 mg/L

  B.   30 mg/L

  C.   20 mg/L

  D.   10 mg/L

5-55. For best deposition in the lower airways, aerosol particles should be in which size range?

  A.   >10 microns

  B.   5–10 microns

  C.   2–4 microns

  D.   <1 micron

5-56. Which of the following are correct concerning artificial noses?

  A.   they perform auto-humidification by the patient

  B.   they easily deliver 100% RH at body temperature

  C.   their use for extended periods of time is well documented

  D.   all of the above

  E.   A and B only

6

Airway and Suction Equipment

INTRODUCTION

Artificial airways are available from many manufacturers and come in many styles, shapes, and sizes. There is much to know concerning their use and function. Likewise, suction machines and catheters vary considerably. The following exercises will allow review of the information presented in Chapter 6 of *Respiratory Care Equipment*.

Laboratory Exercises

6-1. Using a manikin, demonstrate proper technique for establishment of an airway in an unconscious victim.

6-2. Using a manikin, demonstrate the proper technique for insertion and securing of each of the following: oropharyngeal airway, nasopharyngeal airway, oral endotube, nasal endotube, and esophageal airway.

6-3. Obtain several different laryngoscope handles and blades and perform the following:
    1. Compare and classify their construction.
    2. Disassemble and correctly reassemble each.
    3. Demonstrate proper use of each for intubation.

6-4. Obtain several endotracheal (ET) and tracheostomy tubes and identify all markings and structures present.

6-5. Obtain a syringe and practice inflating and deflating the cuff.

6-6. Obtain appropriate equipment and practice measuring ET tube cuff pressure.

6-7. Using an intubated artificial trachea and positive pressure ventilation, practice creation of the minimal leak and minimal occluding volume techniques.

Clinical Problem Solving: Student Exercise

For each of the following situations, diagnose the problem and take appropriate action to correct it:

6-8. While working a night shift at a local hospital, you are called to the room of a patient who just suffered a cardiac arrest. While ventilating the patient with a bag-valve-mask (BVM) device, it becomes increasingly difficult to squeeze the bag. There are decreased breath sounds and the abdomen seems to be enlarging.

6-9. A patient has an oropharyngeal airway (bite block) placed appropriately. Shortly afterward, the patient is found gagging with the bite block coming out.

6-10. A cardiac arrest victim has an esophageal obturator airway (EOA) inserted and ventilation is begun. On assessment, no breath sounds are found and the abdomen is distending.

6-11. An adult patient, whose history is unknown, is newly intubated with an ET tube. Breath sounds are present on the right side of the thorax but not on the left.

6-12. Following a difficult nasal intubation using direct laryngeal visualization, 6 mL of air is used to inflate the ET tube cuff. When attempting to ventilate, a large gas leakage is heard coming from around the tube. Another 6 mL of air is injected into the cuff, but the leak persists.

6-13. While attempting to intubate a patient, it is discovered that the light does not function on the laryngoscope blade.

6-14. A patient needs an emergency intubation. How do you determine the appropriate size ET tube for intubation?

6-15. An intubated, mechanically ventilated patient has just returned from the OR. You want to evaluate the appropriateness of the cuff pressure but a manometer is not available. You squeeze the pilot balloon and find it to be very stiff (hard).

6-16. An intubated patient on a mechanical ventilator has a large leak around the ET tube cuff at 20 mm Hg (27 cm H_2O). In an attempt to create a seal, the pressure is increased to 30 mm Hg (41 cm H_2O). At this pressure, a moderate leak still occurs. X-ray has determined that the tube is positioned properly. You notice that the tube size is rather small for the patient's size. Is the patient in danger of tracheal damage from the elevated cuff pressure?

Research Projects

1. Design a project to measure the pressure exerted against the tracheal wall by an inflated cuff at different cuff pressures and with different size ET tubes. Compare the pressure measured at the cuff–trachea interface to the pressure measured inside the cuff.
2. According to Poiseuille's law, resistance to flow is directly related to the length of a tube and inversely related to a tube's diameter. Design a study to measure back-pressure and calculate resistance with various tube lengths and sizes at different flow rates.

ET TUBE AND SUCTION CATHETER SIZE

Endotracheal tubes come in many sizes, with each tube having its size printed on its side. Actually, several size values may be printed on a tube: the OD or outer diameter, which is the external diameter of the tube in millimeters, and the ID or inner diameter, which is the internal diameter of the tube in millimeters. When stating the size of the tube used to intubate a patient, the ID is the number quoted. This number can also be located on the 15-mm endotracheal tube adapter used for connection to mechanical ventilator circuits or Briggs' adapters. This allows tube size documentation after intubation, if it was not noted prior to intubation.

Another measurement, the FR or French size of the tube, is the external circumference of the tube in millimeters. The circumference (*C*) of a circle is equal to the diameter (*D*) of the circle times π. The Greek letter π is pronounced "pie" and is approximately equal to 3.14. This is expressed in the following formula:

$$C = D \times \pi$$

If either the C or D is known, the other can be calculated. These values are important in selecting the appropriate size tube for intubation. Likewise, knowledge of ET tube size is important in selecting the appropriate size suction catheter.

Calculation of Appropriate Catheter Size for ET Suctioning: The 2/3 Rule

It has been suggested that a catheter for ET suctioning be selected according to the following rule:

> The external diameter of the suction catheter
> should not be more than two-thirds of the internal
> diameter of the ET tube, "the 2/3 rule."

Suction catheters are classified by French sizes (8, 10, 12, 14, 16, etc.), with each size referring to the external circumference of the catheter in millimeters. Using the above information, the appropriate size suction catheter can be determined for any ET tube size by comparing the external suction catheter diameter with the internal diameter of the ET tube. In the following examples, π will be allowed to equal 3.

Example
Using the 2/3 rule, calculate the maximum size suction catheter recommended for use with a #8 ET tube? The ID of a #8 tube is 8 mm.
- Two-thirds of this value is 5.3 mm ($2/3 \times 8 = 5.3$).
- This means that the largest suction catheter to be used must not have an external diameter of more than 5.3 mm.
- By using the formula $C = \pi \times D$, the appropriate catheter size can be determined.
  $C = 3 \times 5.3$ or
  $C = 15.9$, rounded off to 16
- This calculation yields an answer of 16. Thus, a 16 FR catheter, which has an external diameter of 5.3 mm, is the largest suction catheter to be used with a #8 ET tube.
- A simpler calculation is to multiply the ET tube size times 2 ($8 \times 2 = 16$). Again, this follows the 2/3 rule and results in a number which reflects the maximum French size suction catheter that is recommended for use with any ET tube.

Calculation of Appropriate Catheter Size for ET Suctioning: The 1/2 Rule

It also has been suggested that the suction catheter should not have an external diameter larger than one-half the internal diameter of the ET tube, "the 1/2 rule."

> The external diameter of the suction catheter
> should not be more than one-half the internal
> diameter of the ET tube, "the 1/2 rule."

Selection of suction catheters by the 1/2 rule is highly recommended by this author for decreasing some of the hazards associated with ET suctioning.

Example

What is the maximum size suction catheter recommended for use with a #8 ET tube? The ID of a #8 tube is 8 mm.

- One-half of this value is 4 mm ($.5 \times 8 = 4$).
- This means that the largest suction catheter to be used must not have an external diameter of more than 4 mm.
- By using the formula $C = \pi \times D$, the appropriate catheter size can be determined.
    $C = 3 \times 4$ or $C = 12$
- This calculation yields an answer of 12. Thus, a 12 FR catheter, which has an external diameter of 4 mm, is the largest suction catheter to be used with a #8 ET tube.
- A simpler calculation is to multiply the ET tube size times 1.5 ($8 \times 1.5 = 12$). Again, this follows the 1/2 rule, and results in a number which reflects the maximum French size suction catheter that is recommended for use with any ET tube.

SUCTION PRESSURE REGULATION

As mentioned in *Respiratory Care Equipment*, there are many suction regulators or devices that can be used to create subambient pressure. Regardless of the device utilized, it must be regulated and monitored to avoid some of the hazards associated with suctioning. Although subambient pressures quoted as being appropriate for suctioning may vary from author to author, the following are recommended here. For infants use –60 to –80 mm Hg; for children use –80 to –100 mm Hg; and for adults use –100 to –120 mm Hg. There are times when pressures exceeding these parameters will be needed. It is best to use the lowest pressure that is still effective for clearing secretions. Review the conversions to inches of Hg and cm H_2O since some suction devices may also be calibrated using these pressure units.

Critical Thinking Exercises

6-17. Generate a list of 8–10 different complications associated with endotracheal suctioning. Generate a second list of methods used to help prevent these complications.

6-18. What are the largest size suction catheters recommended for use with the following ET tube sizes?

	ET Tube Size	(2/3 rule) Suction Catheter	(1/2 rule) Suction Catheter
a.	10	_____	_____
b.	9	_____	_____
c.	8	16 FR	12 FR
d.	7	_____	_____
e.	6	_____	_____
f.	5	_____	_____
g.	4	_____	_____
h.	3	_____	_____

Laboratory Exercises

6-19. Compare the following vacuum systems: central vacuum, portable suction pump, and venturi suction. Practice making pressure adjustments for different levels of suction pressure required.

6-20. Obtain several types of suction catheters including a curved tip catheter and a closed system suctioning set-up. Compare the catheters and demonstrate proper suctioning technique with each.

Research Projects

1. Design a project to measure the amount of volume removed by a suction catheter during suctioning. Set up a known volume of gas (maybe using a water seal spirometer, a plastic bag, or test lung with a known volume of gas). Intubate the container and measure the amount of air removed from it by using different size suction catheters, at different suction pressures, for varying amounts of time, and with different size ET tubes.

2. Design a project to measure the amount of subambient (negative) pressure generated inside a test lung when varying the size of the suction catheter, the size of the ET tube, the suction pressure used, and the time during which the suction is applied.

REVIEW QUESTIONS

6-21. Which of the following is most desirable for a patient who would require only periodic tracheal suctioning?
 A.   a trach button
 B.   a Jackson metal trach tube
 C.   an uncuffed plastic trach tube
 D.   a fenestrated trach tube

6-22. Which of the following is/are examples of a double-lumen endotracheal tube?
  I.   Carlens
  II.   Whyte
  III.   Cole
  IV.   Rae
 A.   I only
 B.   I and II only
 C.   II and III only
 D.   I and IV only

6-23. When using the straight blade of a laryngoscope, where is the blade tip to be placed?
 A.   into the trachea
 B.   into the vallecula, lifting the epiglottis indirectly
 C.   against the epiglottis, lifting it directly
 D.   into the oropharyngeal area

6-24. Which "plastic" is most commonly used for manufacture of ET tubes?
 A.   teflon
 B.   polyethylene
 C.   polyvinylchloride
 D.   silicon

6-25. The standard laryngoscope and blade is designed to be held in _____ during intubation?

A. the right hand
B. the left hand
C. either hand

6-26. Magill forceps would most likely be used during which of the following procedures?
A. tracheostomy
B. nasotracheal intubation
C. orotracheal intubation
D. extubation

6-27. The main function of the obturator used with a tracheostomy tube or naso-pharyngeal tube is to:
A. facilitate tube insertion
B. remove dried secretions
C. aid in suctioning
D. aid in decannulation

6-28. The primary advantage of a fenestrated tracheostomy tube is that it:
A. reduces the incident of tracheal injury
B. reduces mucus production
C. reduces nosocomial infections
D. facilitates communication

6-29. Advantages of artificial airways that have a large residual cuff volume over the "high pressure" cuffs include:
I. a lower cuff–tracheal wall pressure
II. a better cuff–tracheal seal
III. greater protection against aspiration
IV. less likely cuff tear during insertion
A. I only
B. I and III only
C. I, II, and III only
D. I, II, and IV only

6-30. While performing a ventilator check, it is discovered that a small leak around the ET tube cuff occurs during peak pressure of the sigh breath. The cuff is inflated to 20 mm Hg. What is the most appropriate action?
A. increase the cuff pressure until the leak stops
B. decrease the cuff pressure to 15 mm Hg
C. suggest a larger ET tube be used to replace the present ET tube
D. leave the situation as it is

6-31. Which of the following are potential complications with usage of an EOA?
I. tracheal intubation
II. gastric distention
III. a ruptured esophagus
IV. unilateral lung inflation
A. I and II only
B. I, II, and III only
C. II, III, and IV only
D. I, II, III, and IV

6-32. While attempting to perform ET suctioning on a patient, the therapist is unable to clear the thick secretions. The ET tube is a #7, the suction catheter is a FR 14, and

the suction pressure is set at –80 mm Hg. Which of the following actions is the most appropriate?
A. obtain a FR 16 suction catheter
B. replace the suction regulator
C. increase the suction pressure to –120 mm Hg
D. attach the suction tubing directly to the ET tube

6-33. The device best suited to help prevent short-term upper airway obstruction in a conscious patient who does not require mechanical ventilation is the:
A. oropharyngeal airway
B. nasopharyngeal airway
C. trach button
D. orotracheal tube

6-34. Overinflation of the cuff of an ET tube would most likely result in
A. decreased local capillary blood flow
B. laryngospasm
C. decreased lung compliance
D. increased airway resistance

6-35. The most appropriate means to maintain a patent airway in an unconscious patient who is not intubated is to:
A. sit the patient up
B. place a pillow under the head
C. perform the head tilt/chin lift maneuver
D. place the patient in the prone position

6-36. Which of the following are appropriate for helping to determine proper ET tube placement?
I. chest X-ray
II. auscultation of the epigastrium
III. auscultation of the chest bilaterally
IV. observing the depth markings on the ET tube
A. I and III only
B. I, III, and IV only
C. I, II, and III only
D. I, II, III, and IV

6-37. Ideally, tracheal tube cuff pressures should not exceed:
A. 10 mm Hg
B. 15 mm Hg
C. 20 mm Hg
D. 25 mm Hg

6-38. Appropriate suction pressures for adult patients should be in the subambient range of:
A. 60 to 80 mm Hg
B. 80 to 100 mm Hg
C. 100 to 120 mm Hg
D. 120 to 140 mm Hg

6-39. 20 mm Hg is equal to approximately how many cm H_2O?
A. 37
B. 27
C. 20
D. 14

7

Manual and Gas-Powered Resuscitators

INTRODUCTION

Resuscitators, bag–valve (B–V) or bag–valve–mask (B–V–M) units, mouth-to-mask devices, face shields, and other barrier devices are important when performing rescue breathing so that mouth-to-mouth ventilation does not need to be performed. In many cases, the use of resuscitation devices allows appropriate volume delivery at an appropriate respiratory rate while incorporating delivery of supplemental O_2. Although much research has been done on B–V devices, manufacturers are constantly producing new and updated models. These devices, along with other resuscitation units, need to be evaluated. Features to be evaluated include: volume delivery, valve resistance, FIO_2 delivery, cost, size and portability, ease of use, protection of rescuer from victim's exhaled gas and secretions, application to various sized victims, durability, and operation under adverse conditions such as extremes of temperature.

Laboratory Exercises

Listed below are a few suggestions for studies that are easy to perform and are needed for product evaluation. These studies may result in publishable material. All three types of units—adult, pediatric, and infant—should be evaluated.

7-1   *Volume delivery:* Using a resuscitator bag, a volume measuring device which can be attached to the bag, and a test lung, measure the volumes that can be delivered under varying conditions such as:
   • one hand squeezing the bag
   • two hands squeezing the bag
   • test lung with a low compliance
   • test lung with a high compliance
   • test lung with a low resistance to breathing
   • test lung with a high resistance to breathing

7-2   *Volume delivery:* Using a manikin for rescue breathing, measure the actual volume delivered under various conditions with different devices:

- using different face shields
- using different mouth-to-mask devices
- using different bag–valve–mask units with one person and two persons manipulating the bag and mask

7-3. *FIO$_2$ delivery*: Using different resuscitation devices and an O$_2$ analyzer, determine the FIO$_2$ delivered by these devices under varying conditions. These may include:
- changing the O$_2$ flow rate
- changing the tidal volume (stroke volume) delivered from a bag–valve
- changing the respiratory rate
- use of a reservoir that varies in size
- manually restricting the recoil of the bag, thus increasing the time allowed for the resuscitator bag to fill with gas

7-4. *Pressure release or pop-off setting*: Using various bag–valve devices, a test lung, and a pressure measuring device adapted into the system, measure the pressure at which the pop-off opens, releasing excess pressure into the atmosphere. Compare it to the manufacturer's stated setting.

7-5. *Back-pressure and resistance to flow*: Using various resuscitation devices and a pressure measuring device, measure the back-pressure generated when a given flow rate of gas is passed through the valve. The resistance to flow can be calculated by dividing the back-pressure by the flow rate in liters per second. This can be checked for both inspiratory and expiratory flow rates when applicable.

7-6. *Respiratory rate*: Using different bag–valve units and a test lung, attempt to ventilate the test lung very rapidly. Allow the bag to completely fill before squeezing it again. Record the rate.

7-7. *O$_2$-powered resuscitators*: According to published guidelines, O$_2$-powered resuscitators are to be limited to a flow of 40 L/min and a pressure limit of 60 cm H$_2$O. Select several O$_2$-powered resuscitators along with a flow measuring device and a pressure measuring device and perform an evaluation of proper operation.

7-8. Select a variety of bag–valve devices. Dismantle each one and inspect the inlet valve for method of operation. Inspect the patient valve connector for operation during inspiration and exhalation. Reassemble the units.

Clinical Problem Solving: Student Exercise

For each of the following situations, diagnose the problem and take appropriate action to correct it.

7-9. While attempting to ventilate a patient with a bag–valve resuscitator, the bag can be squeezed very easily and air is felt exiting the bag at the air inlet valve.

7-10. While attempting to ventilate a patient, the resuscitator bag refills with gas very slowly.

7-11. After being called to the room of a patient requiring CPR, a bag–valve device is obtained and ventilation is begun. The device has no O_2 reservoir. How can the FIO_2 be optimized in this situation?

REVIEW QUESTIONS

7-12. One of the most common complications to occur when using a B–V–M is:
   A. pneumothorax
   B. subcutaneous emphysema
   C. laryngospasm
   D. gastric insufflation

7-13. The O_2 delivered by a B–V–M is dependent on all of the following except:
   A. flow rate of O_2
   B. bag refill time
   C. mean airway pressure
   D. manual ventilation rate

7-14. A patient requires manual/mechanical ventilation. Which of the following would deliver the highest FIO_2?
   A. a non-rebreathing mask
   B. an O_2-powered resuscitator
   C. a B–V–M with O_2 at 10 L/min but without a reservoir
   D. a B–V–M with O_2 at 10 L/min but with a reservoir

7-15. The mask for mouth-to-mask ventilation should:
   A. have the standard 15/22 mm connector
   B. have a relatively large dead space
   C. be opaque
   D. all of the above
   E. A and B only

7-16. The primary purpose of a filter in a mouth-to-mask device is to:
   A. protect the rescuer
   B. protect the victim
   C. protect bystanders
   D. filter the incoming flow of O_2 from the O_2 source

7-17. Which of the following are correct?
   I. lower volumes are delivered with the use of one hand as compared to two hands when using a B–V device

II. increased lung impedance tends to decrease volumes delivered by a B–V device

III. fatigue is not a factor affecting volume delivery with a B–V device for short periods of time

IV. operator skill does affect volume delivery when using a B–V device

A. I and II only
B. I and III only
C. II, III, and IV only
D. I, II, III, and IV

7-18. With flow-inflating resuscitator bags, the end expiratory pressure in the bag is controlled by which of the following?

A. the O_2 flow into the bag
B. the bleed-off rate
C. the pressure release (pop-off) setting
D. all of the above
E. A and B only

7-19. The "ideal" manual resuscitator should have which of the following characteristics?

I. a standard 15/22 mm adapter
II. a rapid recoil so high ventilatory rates can be used if necessary
III. deliver any desired FIO_2
IV. have a non-rebreathing valve

A. I and II only
B. I and III only
C. II, III, and IV only
D. I, II, III, and IV

7-20. Regarding the use of B–V resuscitators, which of the following are correct during single rescuer use?

A. it is difficult to prevent leaks around the mask with one hand
B. it is difficult to maintain a patent airway with one hand
C. it is easy to deliver the recommended volume with one hand
D. all of the above
E. A and B only

7-21. The AHA recommends what minimal volume delivery from a B–V device during manual ventilation?

A. 600 mL
B. 800 mL
C. 1000 mL
D. 1200 mL

7-22. Which of the following statements are correct concerning oxygen-powered resuscitators?

A. they deliver 100% oxygen
B. the pressure delivered by the device should be limited to 60 cm H_2O
C. the flow rate delivered by the device should be limited to 40 L/min
D. all of the above
E. A and B only

8

Blood Gases: The Measurement of pH, PCO2, PO2, and Related Analytes

INTRODUCTION

Arterial blood sampling via arterial puncture is probably the most common invasive procedure performed by RCPs. For those learning the technique, it can also be one of the most challenging. Like many other areas of respiratory care, the equipment used for obtaining and analyzing blood samples has undergone much change in the past 20 years. The era of routinely obtaining blood samples without protective equipment (gloves) is past. The number of different models of syringes available for performing arterial punctures would rival the variety of cereals found in a grocery store. Labor intensive analyzers have been replaced with automated machines that require relatively little manual labor.

Chapter 8 presents a discussion of the electrodes used in analyzers, the calibration of analyzers, and quality control procedures used for verifying analyzer results.

HEMOGLOBIN AND HEMATOCRIT

Under normal conditions total hemoglobin (tHb) and hematocrit (Hct) have a relationship expressed in the following formula:

$$tHb \times 3 \approx Hct$$

where
  tHb is in grams of Hb/100 mL of blood, or deciliter of blood (dL)
  tHb may also be expressed as g%
  Hct is the % packed red blood cells by volume in a blood sample

This formula represents an approximation, and such a relationship between hemoglobin and hematocrit will not be valid in certain hematologic disorders.

Example

A patient with a tHb of 14 g% will have an approximate Hct of 42% (3 × 14). Likewise, a patient with a Hct of 39% will have an approximate tHb of 13 g% (39/3).

TEMPERATURE CORRECTION

Blood gas values are routinely measured and reported at 37°C. It is important that the temperature of the analyzer always be maintained at 37°C. This is relatively easy. The patient, however, may not always be so easy to maintain at 37°C. Whether or not the values obtained from a patient whose temperature is not at 37°C will be corrected to 37°C depends on the policy at the institution. If the patient's temperature is less than 37°C, the gas values reported at 37°C will be higher than they actually are in the patient's body. The pH, however, will be lower. If the patient's temperature is higher than 37°C, the opposite will be true for gas and pH values. The following example portrays this relationship. The numbers used here are for illustration only.

Example

A patient was brought to the hospital after suffering cold exposure during the night. His core body temperature was 34°C. An arterial blood gas was performed and the results, at 37°C, were as follows: pH = 7.30, P_{CO_2} = 46 torr, and P_{O_2} = 85 torr. When corrected to 34°C, the values would look like this: pH = 7.35, P_{CO_2} = 39 torr, and P_{O_2} = 65 torr.

Manual calculations such as these can be done, but the correction is routinely performed by the ABG analyzer. However, it is necessary for the operator to key the machine to make a temperature adjustment.

FRACTIONAL VERSUS FUNCTIONAL HEMOGLOBIN

Fractional Hemoglobin

Fractional oxyhemoglobin (FO_2Hb) is the amount of oxyhemoglobin (O_2Hb) expressed as a fraction of the total hemoglobin (tHb). tHb includes all forms of Hb.

$$FO_2Hb = O_2Hb/tHb$$

where $tHb = O_2Hb + HHb + COHb + MetHb + \cdots$.

Functional Hemoglobin

Functional oxygen saturation, or oxygen saturation of available hemoglobin (SO_2), is the amount of oxyhemoglobin—expressed as a fraction of the Hb—which has the ability to bind with oxygen. This includes only oxyhemoglobin (O_2Hb) and deoxyhemoglobin (HHb). Sometimes HHb is also referred to as reduced Hb.

$$SO_2 = O_2Hb/(O_2Hb + HHb)$$

At times, a patient's FO_2Hb and SO_2 values may be very similar; at others, they may be quite different.

Examples

Example 1
A patient has the following Hb levels:

Hb levels	fraction of tHb	% of tHb
tHb = 15.0 g	1.0	100
O_2Hb = 14.4 g	0.96	96
COHb = 0.15 g	0.01	1
MetHb = 0.15 g	0.01	1
HHb = 0.3 g	0.02	2

$FO_2Hb = 14.4/15 = .96$ or 96%
$SO_2 = 14.4/14.7 = .98$ or 98%

Example 2
A patient has the following Hb levels:

Hb levels	fraction of tHb	% of tHb
tHb = 15.0 g	1.0	100
O_2Hb = 12.75 g	0.85	85
COHb = 1.5 g	0.1	10
MetHb = 0.45 g	0.03	3
HHb = 0.30 g	0.02	2

$FO_2Hb = 12.75/15 = .85$ or 85%
$SO_2 = 12.75/13.05 = .98$ or 98%

In Example 1, the two saturation values are very similar. In Example 2, there is a great difference in the reported values. If the co-oximeter in use allows a choice between fractional and functional Hb read-outs, choose the fractional setting. It gives a truer picture of the amount of O_2 actually present and available on the Hb. It will also alert operators when there is a problem with the saturation of the hemoglobin without calling up the other Hb values.

Laboratory Exercises

8-1. Spend time operating, calibrating, and, in general, becoming familiar with a blood gas analyzer.

8-2. Blood gas analyzers can also measure the PO_2 and PCO_2 values in a gaseous sample. Inject a room air sample into the analyzer. Record the results. Are they the same as the predicted results? (Remember that the analyzer is calibrated to BTPS)

8-3. Inject a 100% oxygen gas sample into the analyzer. Record the results. Are they the same as predicted?

8-4. Bubble 100% oxygen through water. Aspirate a water sample into a syringe and measure the Po_2 in the blood gas analyzer.

REVIEW QUESTIONS

8-5. While caring for a patient, the following blood gases are obtained: pH = 7.05, Paco_2 = 15 torr, HCO$_3-$ = 4 mEq/L, and Pao_2 = 120 torr. What is the most likely conclusion drawn from this data?
A. The patient is breathing supplemental O$_2$
B. The patient has a compensated metabolic acidemia
C. The patient has a normal blood gas
D. The patient is hyperventilating due to an acid–base disturbance

8-6. While calibrating a blood gas analyzer with a calibrating gas of 10% O$_2$, the Po_2 reading should be set at what value if the barometric pressure is 760 torr?
A. 760.0
B. 149.9
C. 76.0
D. 71.3

8-7. The Pao_2 value on an arterial blood gas report is routinely obtained by which method of analysis?
A. paramagnetism
B. polarographic determination
C. thermal conductivity
D. spectrophotometry

8-8. The metals incorporated into a Clark electrode are commonly of which type?
  I. platinum
  II. bronze
  III. gold
  IV. silver
A. I and II only
B. I and IV only
C. II and III only
D. I and IV only

8-9. pH is best defined as:
A. the [H$^+$] active in a solution
B. the log of [H$^+$] active in a solution
C. the negative log of the [H$^+$] active in a solution
D. the total nanomole concentration of [H$^+$] active in a solution

8-10. A blood sample is taken from a patient with a temperature of 39°C. The results analyzed at 37°C are as follows: pH = 7.40, Paco_2 = 40 torr, and Pao_2 = 90 torr. Which of the following would most appropriately approximate the actual values at 39°C?

    A.   pH = 7.45, $PaCO_2$ = 34, PaO_2 = 75
    B.   pH = 7.45, $PaCO_2$ = 34, PaO_2 = 105
    C.   pH = 7.35, $PaCO_2$ = 46, PaO_2 = 75
    D.   pH = 7.35, $PaCO_2$ = 46, PaO_2 = 105

8-11. Measurement of tHb is based on which of the following?
    A.   absorption of light
    B.   paramagnetism
    C.   thermal conductivity
    D.   mass spectrometry

8-12. A "salt bridge" is incorporated for use in which blood gas parameter measurement?
    A.   pH
    B. PCO_2
    C. PO_2
    D. O_2 Saturation

8-13. Protein build-up in the pH electrode will cause which of the following?
    A.   increased responsiveness
    B.   decreased responsiveness
    C.   no change in responsiveness

8-14. The Severinghaus electrode refers to which of the following?
    A.   the CO_2 electrode
    B.   the O_2 electrode
    C.   the pH electrode
    D.   the Na^+ electrode

8-15. The PaO_2 reading on a blood gas analyzer is actually:
    A.   the number of molecules of O_2 present in the sample
    B.   the partial pressure of O_2 in the sample
    C.   the number of O_2 molecules that diffused into the electrode
    D.   the measurement of current flow between the anode and cathode in the electrode

8-16. Quality assurance for ABG analysis could be obtained by use of
    A.   tonometry
    B.   commercially available controls
    C.   duplicate analysis of samples
    D.   all of the above
    E.   A and B only

8-17. Beer's law is used in the measurement of which of the following parameters?
    A.   pH
    B. PCO_2
    C. PO_2
    D. O_2 Sat.

8-18. Potential substances interfering with the co-oximeter readings may include:
    I.   lipids in the blood sample
    II.   dyes in the blood
    III.   deoxyhemoglobin
    IV.   carboxyhemoglobin

A.   I and II only
B.   III and IV only
C.   I, II, and IV only
D.   II, III, and IV only

8-19. Which of the following electrodes are potentiometric, that is, they measure voltage?
A.   pH
B.   PCO_2
C.   PO_2
D.   all of the above
E.   A and B only

8-20. Which of the following are correct concerning the pH electrode?
A.   it is composed in part of pH sensitive glass
B.   it should be maintained at 37°C
C.   it should be in an anaerobic chamber
D.   all of the above
E.   A and B only

8-21. The measurement of which of the following parameters is an adoption of the pH measurement?
A. K^+
B. Na^+
C. O_2
D. CO_2

8-22. Which of the following are correct concerning end point detection during blood gas analysis?
A.   it is the observation that an electrode response is no longer changing
B.   a microprocessor can determine electrical end point
C.   manual end point determination is not possible
D.   all of the above
E.   A and B only

8-23. Levey-Jennings charts help document:
A.   PO_2/hemoglobin relations
B.   quality control results over time
C.   acid–base ratios
D.   all of the above
E.   A and B only

8-24. Two common types of materials used for the membranes of the CO_2 electrode are:
I.   silastic
II.   teflon
III. nylon
IV.   polypropylene
A.   I and II only
B.   I and III only
C.   II and III only
D.   II and IV only
E.   III and IV only

8-25. The number of electrons needed to reduce each molecule of O_2 in the O_2 electrode is:
   A.   one
   B.   two
   C.   three
   D.   four

8-26. For the correct measurement of a patient's hemoglobin level, which of the following must occur?
   A.   the system must be calibrated correctly
   B.   the sample must be well mixed
   C.   complete hemolysis must have occurred
   D.   all of the above
   E.   A and B only

8-27. A patient is found to have a Hct of 25. What would be the estimated Hb value?
   A.   75 g%
   B.   25 g%
   C.   8.3 g%
   D.   4.8 g%

8-28. What is the fractional oxyhemoglobin (FO_2Hb) concentration (in %) for a patient with the following Hb levels?
   tHb = 10 g, O_2Hb = 8 g,   COHb = 1 g,   MetHb = 0.5 g,   and   HHb = 0.5 g.
   A.   100%
   B.   94%
   C.   80%
   D.   75%

8-29. What is the functional oxyhemoglobin saturation (SO_2) in a patient with the following Hb levels?
   tHb = 10 g, O_2Hb = 8 g,   COHb = 1 g,   MetHb = 0.5 g,   and   HHb = 0.5 g.
   A.   100%
   B.   94%
   C.   80%
   D.   75%

9

Noninvasive Respiratory Monitoring Equipment

INTRODUCTION

Chapter 9 presents information on various types of monitoring equipment. Included in the discussion are oxygen analyzers, pulse oximeters, capnometers, mass spectrometers, calorimeters, and equipment for measuring waveforms during mechanical ventilation.

OXYGEN ANALYZERS

There are many models of O_2 analyzers, and some common principles can be applied to most. Polarographic analyzers need some type of external power source to energize the sensor. This energy may come from the direct current (DC) of batteries or from 110 volts alternating current (AC) of wall outlets. This energy would also be used to operate the alarms, digital readouts, etc., associated with the analyzer. Galvanic analyzers do not need a power source for sensor operation but will need an energy source if alarms, digital readouts, etc., are part of the device. Both of these analyzer types measure PO_2 yet the readout is often calibrated in FO_2 or $O_2\%$ which is calculated from the PO_2 reading. This is why an analyzer reads lower if taken to a higher altitude. This occurs even though the actual FIO_2 remains at 21%. However, because the total pressure is lower, the PO_2 drops, and the reading on the analyzer also drops below 21%. This concept tends to create confusion among individuals who are unfamiliar with the devices. These analyzers can report accurate results if they are recalibrated at the altitude at which they are used.

Calibration of Oxygen Analyzers

Special attention should be given to the calibration of O_2 analyzers. Although some O_2 analyzers have a two-point calibration (a high and low value), most portable analyzers have what is called a one-point calibration. That is, they are calibrated to room air (21% O_2) **or** to 100% O_2. In reality, they can be calibrated to any FIO_2 if a known percent oxygen gas source is available. Manufacturers recommend, however, that analyzers be calibrated to 100%. As long as the reading returns to approximately 21% when exposed to room air, it is operating correctly. If the reading does not return to approximately 21%, the sensor may need to be replaced.

Some manufacturers state that it is satisfactory to calibrate at 21%, but this is less than ideal. Calibrating at 21% will more likely result in a greater % error when analyzing O_2, especially at the high O_2 concentrations. Occasionally it is recommended that analyzers be calibrated to the appropriate concentration of gases to be analyzed. If this is less than 60% oxygen, calibrate at 21%. If it is equal to or greater than 60% oxygen, calibrate at 100%.

The typical calibration procedure for analog meters (devices with an indicator needle) is as follows:

- place the analyzer in the standby mode
- use the *zero control screw* to set the analyzer indicator to zero. This is an electronic zero of the meter. This zeroing is important, but is not really part of the one-point calibration. Digital meters do not require a manual zeroing; it is done automatically.
- after zeroing, with the analyzer turned on, and the sensor exposed to a known O_2 concentration, use the *calibrate screw or knob* to adjust the indicator to the appropriate value. If in 21% oxygen, adjust it to 21%. If in 100% oxygen, adjust it to 100%.

This is the one-point calibration. Calibrating at one end of the scale does not mean the other end of the scale will come in at the exact concentration. However, if the sensor is in good working order, it will be close. An analyzer, which has a one-point calibration (one calibration knob), cannot be calibrated at both ends of the scale. That procedure is a two-point calibration and is unavailable on a one-point calibration device. An analyzer may be accurate over the entire scale, but it is not due to the ability to dial in both ends of the scale. Please consult the manufacturer's directions for the proper calibration procedure for the oxygen analyzer being utilized.

Laboratory Exercise

9-1.   Obtain one or more oxygen analyzers and perform the following: Observe the construction and method of operation. Determine the units used on the readout scale. Calibrate the analyzer following the manufacturer's guidelines. Set alarm limits if applicable. Analyze a gas sample.

Critical Thinking Exercises

9-2.   A galvanic O_2 analyzer is being used to analyze the FIO_2 delivered from a ventilator. The analyzer utilizes drying crystals to remove humidity from the sample prior to measuring the PO_2. When placed in the circuit proximal to the humidifier it reads 40%, what will it read when placed distal to the humidifier? (RH = 100% at 37°C)

9-3.   Repeat the situation in 9-2, but this time do not use drying crystals. How will the two readings compare?

9-4. Three O_2 analyzer sensors are placed in-line to measure the FIO_2 delivered from a jet nebulizer. The first one reads 52%, the second one reads 50%, and the third one reads 48% O_2. Assuming all are calibrated correctly, list some reasons why three analyzers may all read differently.

9-5. A jet nebulizer is set up to deliver 40% O_2 following the physician's order. When analyzed, it reads 50%. What steps should be taken to determine the reason for the inconsistency and what should be done to correct it?

9-6. An O_2 analyzer with drying crystals calibrated at 100% is placed in-line in a ventilator circuit where a pressure of 60 cm H_2O is being generated. How may this affect the reading of the O_2 analyzer when the ventilator setting is at 60% O_2?

PULSE OXIMETRY

Pulse oximetry is used to determine the O_2 Saturation (O_2 Sat) of hemoglobin (Hb). Pulse oximetry does not measure pH, $PaCO_2$ or PaO_2. Therefore, it cannot supply information on acid–base status, alveolar ventilation, or PaO_2. PaO_2, however, can be estimated. Or can it?

PaO_2 and O_2 Sat have a relationship expressed by the oxyhemoglobin (O_2Hb) dissociation curve. The graph of this curve, with O_2 Sat on the y-axis and PaO_2 on the x-axis, illustrates this relationship (Figure 9-1). Due to the binding nature of O_2 with Hb, the curve

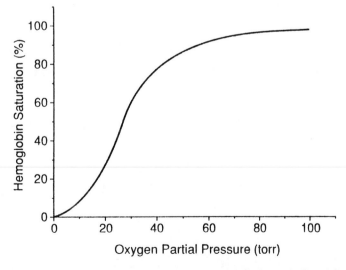

Figure 9-1. Oxyhemoglobin dissociation curve illustrating the relationship between the oxygen partial pressure (PO_2) and the percentage of hemoglobin binding sites that are occupied by oxygen molecules (% sat)

is sigmoid (S) shaped and not a straight line. Many factors can affect the relationship between these two variables. Some of these factors include $PaCO_2$, $[H^+]$ (hydrogen ion concentration), 2,3-diphosphoglycerate (2,3-DPG) levels, and patient temperature.

Increases in all of these factors will shift the curve to the right; decreases in these factors will shift the curve to the left. (Remember that $\uparrow[H^+]$ will $\downarrow$pH.) A right shift means that O_2 will not combine as readily with Hb, but will be released by Hb more easily. A left shift means that O_2 will combine very well with Hb, but will not be released as well.

The actual amount of oxygen released to the tissues depends on many factors, and a blanket statement as to whether a right or left shift is "better" is inappropriate. A right shift results in a lower O_2 Sat for any given PaO_2 when compared to normal. A left shift results in a higher O_2 Sat for any given PaO_2 when compared to normal. For example, normally a PaO_2 of 60 mm Hg will result in an O_2 Sat of approximately 90%. A right shift, with a PaO_2 of 60 mm Hg, would result in a saturation of less than 90%. A left shift, with a PaO_2 of 60 mm Hg, would have a saturation of higher than 90%.

The problem encountered with pulse oximetry is that when measuring only O_2 Sat without the PaO_2 reference value, shifts cannot be determined. A patient can have changes in their PaO_2 along with shifts in the curve. Yet, the O_2 Sat via pulse oximetry cannot reflect this. The significance of this is beyond the scope of this discussion. The point to be emphasized is that the prediction of PaO_2 values from oximetry readings may not be accurate.

Other factors such as abnormal Hb can also interfere with oximetry readings making them totally inaccurate. Carbon monoxide can join with Hb creating carboxyhemoglobin (COHb) which is then unable to bind with O_2. Pulse oximetry interprets COHb as O_2Hb and results in a falsely elevated O_2 Sat reading.

Laboratory Exercise

9-7.   Obtain one or more pulse oximeters and perform the following: Observe the construction and method of operation. Set alarm limits if applicable. Perform a pulse oximetry measurement on a fellow student.

Critical Thinking Exercises

9-8.   A patient is admitted after suffering from smoke inhalation during a house fire. The patient is unharmed except that he was overcome by smoke. In the emergency department, a pulse oximetry measurement is requested. The reading, while the patient is on O_2 via NRM, is 99%. What is the appropriate course of action?

9-9.   A patient with a PaO_2 of 80 mm Hg has an oximetry performed which yields a reading of 92% O_2 Sat. Can this be correct?

Research Project

New models of pulse oximeters are continually being manufactured. Design a study to compare oximetry readings with arterial blood gas (ABG) analysis. Determine accuracy by recording mean values and standard deviation (SD) of the oximeter.

CAPNOMETRY

Capnometry is the measurement of the partial pressure of exhaled CO_2 ($PeCO_2$). The capnograph is a device which displays the waveform of that measurement. *Respiratory Care Equipment* discusses the uses of capnometry, and factors which affect its measurements. Figure 9-27 in *Respiratory Care Equipment* illustrates a normal waveform. Use the information given there to decide what each of the following represent.

Critical Thinking Exercises

9-10. A tracing rises rather quickly and levels off at 60 mm Hg.

9-11. A tracing has a downward spike right in the middle of the exhalation plateau.

9-12. A tracing has a slow rise in exhaled CO_2 and does not plateau.

9-13. A tracing has a series of expiratory plateaus occurring rapidly at 20 mm Hg.

CALORIMETRY

In certain patient populations, it is desirable to know energy expenditure. This can be done by using an equation such as the Harris–Benedict equation which estimates basal energy expenditure (BEE) based on gender, height, weight, and age. Following is the Harris–Benedict equation:

$$BEE = 66 + (13.7 \times W) + (5 \times H) - (6.8 \times A) \quad \text{for males}$$

$$BEE = 65.5 + (9.6 \times W) + (1.7 \times H) - (4.7 \times A) \text{ for females}$$

where
  BEE is basal energy expenditure in kilocalories per day
  W is the weight in kilograms
  H is the height in centimeters
  A is the age in years

Another option is calorimetry, a method used to measure actual resting energy expenditure (REE). Its formula is given below:

$$REE = [(3.94 \times VO_2) + (1.11 \times VCO_2)] \times 1440$$

where
  REE is resting energy in kilocalories per day
  VO_2 is oxygen consumption in liters per minute
  VCO_2 is carbon dioxide production in liters per minute

The following is an example of a patient situation where the two methods of calculating energy expenditure are compared.

Example

A 40-year-old male received chest injuries in a motor vehicle accident. After being stabilized at the scene, he was transported to a local trauma unit. Because he was intubated and unable to eat, caregivers were concerned that he receive the proper nutritional support. The patient weighed 90 kg and was 180 cm tall. An estimate of his calorie requirements using the Harris–Benedict equation resulted in the following:

$$BEE = 66 + (13.7 \times 90) + (5 \times 180) - (6.8 \times 40)$$

$$BEE = 66 + 1233 + 900 - 272 = 1927 \text{ kcal}$$

Due to the extent of his injury, the BEE was increased by a factor of 50% to compensate for the suspected increased metabolic rate. This brought the total estimate to approximately 2890 kcal.

Indirect calorimetry was then performed on the patient. His oxygen consumption (VO_2) was measured at 0.55 L/min and his carbon dioxide production (VCO_2) was measured at 0.48 L/min. Using the Weir equation, the patient's actual calorie requirements were determined.

$$REE = [(3.94 \times 0.55) + (1.11 \times 0.48)] \times 1440$$

$$REE = [2.167 + .533] \times 1440$$

$$REE = 2.70 \times 1440 = 3888 \text{ kcal}$$

In this situation, the patient had other factors increasing his metabolic rate beyond what was predicted. If the patient had received nutritional support according to the estimated need, he would have been underfed by 998 kcal/day.

REVIEW QUESTIONS

9-14. Which of the following would provide the best information concerning oxygen transport to the tissues following smoke inhalation?
   A.   oxygen saturation via pulse oximeter
   B. PaO_2
   C.   measured arterial oxygen content
   D.   tHb concentration

9-15. What is the static compliance of a patient on mechanical ventilation who has a V_t of 800 ml, a peak pressure of 30 cm H_2O, a plateau pressure of 20 cm H_2O, a PEEP of +5 cm H_2O, and an inspiratory flow rate of 40 L/min?
   A.   20.0 mL/cm H_2O
   B.   26.7 mL/cm H_2O
   C.   40.0 mL/cm H_2O
   D.   53.3 mL/cm H_2O
   E.   80.0 mL/cm H_2O

9-16. The capnograph sampling device would be best placed in which of the following sites during mechanical ventilation?
   A.   inspiratory limb of the circuit
   B.   endotracheal tube adapter
   C.   expiratory limb of the circuit
   D.   distal to the exhalation valve

9-17. Which of the following is incorrect concerning the use of a transcutaneous PaO_2 monitor on a neonate?
   A.   room air can be used to calibrate a high point
   B.   a site change should occur two times a day
   C.   probe temperature may be 6–7°C higher than normal body temperature of 37°C
   D.   transcutaneous values should be correlated with arterial values periodically

9-18. Which of the following would not adversely affect the reliability of a capnograph in reporting an appropriate end tidal PCO_2 reading?
   A.   occluded sample line
   B.   a change in the FIO_2
   C.   loose connections in the sampling line
   D.   sample port in the inspiratory line

9-19. Possible causes for being unable to calibrate a galvanic oxygen analyzer include which of the following?
   I.   batteries needing to be replaced
   II.   damaged sensor
   III.   excessive moisture condensed on the sensor
   IV.   calibrating at room temperature

A. I and II only
B. II and III only
C. I, II, and III only
D. II and IV only

9-20. A transcutaneous oxygen reading may be affected by which of the following?
     I.   an air bubble trapped between the membrane and the skin
     II. skin thickness
     III. local tissue perfusion
     IV. skin color
A. I, II, and III only
B. I, II, and IV only
C. I, III, and IV only
D. II and IV only

9-21. Which of the following would be calibrated to zero while the sensor is exposed to room air?
A. galvanic oxygen analyzer
B. transcutaneous oxygen analyzer
C. nitrogen analyzer
D. carbon dioxide analyzer

9-22. Although zeroed appropriately, a galvanic fuel cell oxygen analyzer records only 75% O_2 at maximum gain (the calibration knob is adjusted as far as it goes) in 100% O_2. The appropriate action would be to:
A. change the membrane
B. calibrate to 21% instead of 100%
C. calibrate the sensor under positive pressure conditions
D. replace the fuel cell

9-23. The oxygen analyzer designed on the principle of oxygen being attracted to a magnetic field is called:
A. a zirconium analyzer
B. a calorimeter
C. a paramagnetic analyzer
D. a thermoconductive analyzer

9-24. The type of oxygen analyzer which measures the fractional concentration of oxygen instead of the partial pressure of oxygen is the:
A. paramagnetic
B. electric
C. polarographic
D. electrochemical

9-25. Ideally, airway pressure measurements during mechanical ventilation should take place in which of the following routinely available sites?
A. inspiratory limb (near the machine outlet)
B. expiratory limb (near the expiratory valve)
C. proximal airway (near the patient)

9-26. What is the approximate inspiratory resistance for a patient being mechanically ventilated with a V_t of 800 mL, a peak pressure of 30 cm H_2O, a plateau pressure of 20 cm H_2O, a PEEP of +5 cm H_2O and an inspiratory flow rate of 40 L/min ?
   A.   10 cm H_2O/L/sec
   B.   15 cm H_2O/L/sec
   C.   20 cm H_2O/L/sec
   D.   25 cm H_2O/L/sec
   E.   30 cm H_2O/L/sec

9-27. Following an aerosolized bronchodilator treatment on a mechanically ventilated patient, the pressure–volume loops are widened. This would indicate:
   A.   increased airway resistance
   B.   decreased lung compliance
   C.   decreased work of breathing
   D.   all of the above
   E.   A and B only

9-28. Over a period of time, the pressure–volume loops on a mechanically ventilated patient shift toward the right (decreased slope). This would indicate which of the following?
   A.   increased airway resistance
   B.   decreased lung compliance
   C.   decreased work of breathing
   D.   all of the above
   E.   A and B only

9-29. Increased work of breathing may be due to:
   A.   increased airway secretions
   B.   pulmonary fibrosis
   C.   a small ET tube
   D.   all of the above
   E.   A and B only

9-30. Lung–thorax compliance may be decreased due to:
   A.   atelectasis
   B.   main stem intubation
   C.   abdominal distention
   D.   all of the above
   E.   A and B only

10

Flow and Volume Monitoring Devices

INTRODUCTION

Chapter 10 deals with flow and volume measuring devices. It addresses their general characteristics as well as the standards to which these devices must comply. Many examples of the different types of devices are presented.

Laboratory Exercises

10-1. Using a 3.0-L calibration syringe, test the accuracy and determine the percent error of various volume measuring devices. Compare the results to the manufacturer's specifications. After obtaining proper connectors, inject a known volume of gas through or into a volume measuring device. Conduct tests at varying volumes and flow rates to account for multiple conditions. Some of the devices to be tested include:
    a.   Turbinometers (Wright respirometer)
    b.   Sonic devices (Bear Medical VM-90)
    c.   Bennett spirometer
    d.   Water seal or dry rolling seal spirometers
    e.   Pneumotachometers

The percent error for the device can be calculated by using the following formula:

$$\frac{\text{measured volume} - \text{actual volume}}{\text{actual volume}} \times 100 = \% \text{ error}$$

where the measured volume is the volume recorded by the device and the actual volume is the injected volume of the calibration syringe.

A negative error means the device is recording a volume lower than the actual volume. A positive error means the device is recording a volume higher than the actual volume.

For some of the respirometers (Wright and Bear), make sure that when the volumes are injected into the device, the flow rates stay within the limits of flow for proper function of the device. The Wright respirometer has a flow limit of approximately 3–300 L/min. The Bear VM-90 has a flow limit of approximately 5–250 L/min. Check if the results obtained fall within the acceptable limits given by the manufacturer.

Another factor to be considered is that the calibration syringe contains a volume of gas at ambient conditions. Some of the devices used are calibrated to report the measured volumes at BTPS, others at ambient conditions. This needs to be taken into consideration as percent error is calculated. All volumes must be reported under the same conditions when performing the calculations.

An interesting example of this phenomenon is the Bennett spirometer (BS). Under normal operating conditions, the gas entering the BS is at ATPS, yet it records a volume as if it was at BTPS. If 1.0 L of gas is injected into the BS, it will record approximately 1.1 L. What would the BS record as the volume if 1.0 L of gas, maintained at BTPS, was injected into it? It would record 1.1 L. The spirometer is not designed to detect the fact that the 1.0 L is already at BTPS. It takes whatever volume it receives and makes it appear larger due to its calibration scale.

10-2.   Calculate a bell factor for a spirometer. Using a 3.0 L calibration syringe and a spirometer with a kymograph, paper and pen marker, calculate a bell factor. Set the spirometer volume at 0–2 L. Obtain a baseline tracing with the pen at that setting, then inject 3.0 L of air into the spirometer. After the volume is injected, obtain a new baseline tracing. Using a ruler, measure the length of the line in millimeters resulting from the change in volume. Divide the mm measurement into the volume of 3.0 L.

Examples

Example A

If, after injecting 3.0 L, the line is 75 mm long, the bell factor is calculated by dividing 3000 mL/75 mm, which is 40 mL/mm. This means that for every 1 mm movement of the pen, 40 mL of volume is displaced in the spirometer bellows. The bell factor can now be used to calculate lung volumes based on the pen movement.

Example B

A patient exhales his vital capacity into the spirometer bellows resulting in a line 112 mm long on the kymograph. To determine the volume exhaled, multiply the bell factor times the length of the line—40 mL/mm × 112 mm = 4480 mL or 4.48 L. Remember that this value is at ATPS and needs to be corrected to BTPS by multiplying by the proper BTPS correction factor.

Since most pulmonary function testing (PFT) systems are now computerized, the need to use the bell factor is greatly diminished. However, an understanding of and ability to perform manual calculations on PFT tracings makes the practitioner less hostage to the computer and helps to keep the mind sharp.

REVIEW QUESTIONS

10-3. A portable peak flowmeter consistently records a flow of 90 L/min each time a patient uses the device. Although he states he "feels better" after aerosol treatments, the patient is concerned that he is not getting any better since the peak flow value does not change. The most appropriate action to be taken is:
A. increase the patient's medication dosage
B. admit the patient to the hospital for evaluation
C. recheck the patient's peak flow with another peak flowmeter
D. continue to use the same peak flowmeter for two more weeks

10-4. The fact that a volume measuring device can measure up to 7 L of gas refers to its:
A. accuracy
B. capacity
C. linearity
D. precision

10-5. If an instrument measures the same value as a reference value, it is said to be:
A. accurate
B. durable
C. linear
D. precise

10-6. When an instrument generates reproducible results, it is said to be:
A. accurate
B. certain
C. linear
D. precise

10-7. When an instrument is accurate over the entire range of measurement, it is said to be:
A. certain
B. durable
C. linear
D. precise

10-8. The most appropriate device for documenting accuracy of a water seal spirometer is:
A. a bag–valve device
B. an oxygen flowmeter
C. an air flowmeter
D. a super (calibration) syringe

10-9. When 3 L of air is injected into a rolling seal spirometer from a calibration syringe, the tracing indicates 2.5 L. Which of the following is correct?
A. the difference is within the acceptable percent error
B. the volume was injected too rapidly
C. there is a leak in the system
D. the volume was injected too slowly

10-10. When comparing the FRC measured by the helium dilution technique to the thoracic gas volume (V_{tg}) of the body box in a patient with airflow obstruction, the FRC by helium dilution is often:
A. greater than the V_{tg}
B. less than the V_{tg}
C. the same as the V_{tg}

10-11. Which of the following should be used to detect air flow while performing a sleep study?
A. a capnometer
B. an impedance plethysmograph
C. an esophageal balloon
D. an electrocardiograph

10-12. According to the 1987 ATS standards, a diagnostic spirometer should:
A. have a capacity of at least 7 liters
B. be able to measure flow rates between 0 and 12 L/sec
C. have less than 3% error or measure within 50 mL of a reference value
D. all of the above
E. A and B only

10-13. The length of the pen line on a kymograph, as a result of a VC being performed, is 72 mm. If the bell factor for the spirometer is 43 mL/mm, what is the volume of the VC?
A. 0.6 L
B. 1.7 L
C. 3.1 L
D. 5.9 L

10-14. Turbinometers are not affected by which of the following?
A. temperature
B. turbulence
C. gas composition
D. all of the above
E. A and B only

10-15. The readout from a Fleisch pneumotachometer may be affected by which of the following?
A. condensation
B. turbulent flow
C. gas viscosity
D. all of the above
E. A and B only

11

Pressure Monitoring Devices

INTRODUCTION

Monitoring devices are utilized in many areas of respiratory care. Airway pressure monitoring devices are routinely used with patients receiving mechanical ventilation and other ventilatory support modalities such as CPAP. The devices used for pressure monitoring are described in *Respiratory Care Equipment*. Aneroid manometers have also been discussed in Chapter 3.

REVIEW QUESTIONS

11-1. Force per unit area defines:
   A. gravity
   B. pressure
   C. energy
   D. power

11-2. Mercury is how many times more dense than water?
   A. 0.136
   B. 1.36
   C. 13.6
   D. 136.0

11-3. U-tube type manometers are best for monitoring:
   A. static pressures
   B. dynamic pressures
   C. pressures during mechanical ventilation
   D. pressures during forced exhalation

11-4. The most commonly used pressure manometer in respiratory therapy is:
   A. a gravity dependent manometer
   B. an aneroid manometer
   C. an electromechanical transducer
   D. a piezoelectric device

11-5. A wheatstone bridge circuit is utilized in which type of pressure monitoring device?
A. a gravity dependent manometer
B. an aneroid manometer
C. an electromechanical transducer
D. a piezoelectric device

11-6. A low pressure or disconnect alarm should be set:
A. 5 cm H_2O below the actual pressure
B. 10 cm H_2O below the actual pressure
C. 15 cm H_2O below the actual pressure
D. 20 cm H_2O below the actual pressure

11-7. Airway pressure monitoring devices may digitally display values for:
A. peak inspiratory pressure
B. respiratory frequency
C. tidal volume
D. all of the above
E. A and B only

11-8. Reasons for accidental breathing circuit disconnections may include:
A. inadequate force applied to connections
B. tension on the tubing
C. patient movement
D. all of the above
E. A and B only

11-9. Accidental disconnection of a breathing circuit at the ET tube may elude low pressure alarm detection due to:
A. inappropriate sensor location
B. inappropriate alarm setting
C. a high resistance to flow at the patient connector on the circuit
D. all of the above
E. A and B only

11-10. The mercury barometer is composed of which of the following?
A. a calibrated scale
B. a mercury reservoir
C. a glass tube open at both ends
D. all of the above
E. A and B only

12

Devices for Chest Physiotherapy, Incentive Spirometry, and Intermittent Positive Pressure Breathing

INTRODUCTION

The equipment, and related treatments for which it is used, discussed in this chapter may not always be considered the most exciting aspect of job performance by a respiratory care practitioner. Yet these therapies, and the equipment used to carry them out, are a very important foundation of the profession. These therapies—designed to help in the removal of secretions, the delivery of medications, and the prevention of atelectasis, hypoxemia, and pulmonary infections—are an integral part of the RCP's job duties. Chapter 12 presents the equipment needed to provide these therapies.

Clinical Problem Solving: Student Exercise

For each of the following situations, diagnose the problem and state the appropriate action to be taken to correct the situation.

12-1.   While attempting to perform an incentive spirometry treatment, the practitioner notes that the indicator is registering little volume exchange. The patient appears to be giving a good effort and the chest is expanding with inspiration.

12-2.   While delivering an IPPB treatment with the Bird Mark 7, the practitioner notes that the patient is creating a pressure of −10 cm H_2O before the device cycles on. After cycling to inspiration, the pressure manometer needle remains in the +2 to −2 cm H_2O range until near the end of inspiration. At end inspiration, the needle quickly moves to 20 cm H_2O and the machine cycles off. There is no leak in the system.

12-3.   While attempting to deliver an IPPB treatment with a mouth piece, the device cycles off immediately following initiation of the breath. This happens regardless of the pressure setting.

Laboratory Exercises

12-4.   Set up an IPPB machine and a test lung which has the capability for adjustment of resistance and compliance. Begin with a predetermined baseline setting of flow, pressure, resistance, and compliance. Measure the exhaled gas volume and inspiratory time (T_i). Systematically change the pressure, flow rate, resistance, and compliance one at a time. Document the change in volume and T_i as each change is made. What happens to the T_i and exhaled volume as these changes are made?

12-5.   When powered by 100% oxygen, the venturi in the Bird Mark 7 operates at approximately 40% O_2, if there is no outflow obstruction. This is not the situation during a normal IPPB treatment. Set up a Bird Mark 7 (powered with O_2 and set on air-mix), and a test lung with normal resistance and compliance. Measure the FIO_2 delivered, beginning at low pressures (5 cm H_2O) and then increasing to higher pressures (35 cm H_2O). Allow enough time for stabilization to occur between changes. What happens to the FIO_2 as pressure increases? Why?

12-6.   Obtain both a threshold resistor and a fixed orifice PEP device. Measure the pressures generated while flowing different amounts of gas through the system (10–60 L/min) at a predetermined threshold or orifice setting. Change the threshold or orifice setting and repeat the study. Generate a chart of the pressure measurements as flow increases. Do the two types of devices respond in the same way? (Refer to Chapter 19 for additional information.)

REVIEW QUESTIONS

12-7.   Inspiratory time can be prolonged during an IPPB treatment with a Bird Mark 7 by:
      I.   increasing the pressure setting
      II.   decreasing the pressure setting
      III.   increasing the flow setting
      IV.   decreasing the flow setting
  A.   I and III only
  B.   II and IV only
  C.   II and III only
  D.   I and IV only

12-8.   If a patient has trouble cycling a Bird Mark 7 on to inspiration, the problem likely involves which control?
  A.   sensitivity
  B.   pressure
  C.   flow
  D.   air-mix

12-9.   If a patient complains of dizziness during an incentive spirometry treatment, which of the following is most likely the cause?
  A.   a pneumothorax
  B.   hyperventilation
  C.   carbon dioxide retention
  D.   increased intrathoracic pressure

12-10. What physical change is occurring inside the machine while the pressure setting on the Bird Mark 7 is being increased?
  A.   a pressure transducer is recalibrated
  B.   spring tension is increased
  C.   a magnet and metal plate are brought into closer proximity
  D.   a piston is further compressed into a cylinder

12-11. The pressure displayed on the pressure manometer of the Bird Mark 7 is a measure of the pressure developed:
  A.   in the patient's lungs
  B.   at the patient's mouth
  C.   in the pressure chamber of the Bird
  D.   in the ambient chamber of the Bird

12-12. Chest percussors can be powered by which of the following means?
    A. manually
    B. electrically
    C. pneumatically
    D. all of the above
    E. A and B only

12-13. Incentive spirometers are available in which of the following types?
    A. volume-oriented
    B. flow-oriented
    C. pressure-oriented
    D. all of the above
    E. A and B only

12-14. Indications for IPPB would include:
    A. delivery of medication
    B. secretion removal
    C. lowering $PaCO_2$ levels
    D. all of the above
    E. A and B only

12-15. Although the ceramic valve moves freely on the Bird Mark 7, a patient has difficulty cycling the machine on to inspiration. Which of the following may be responsible?
    A. the pressure magnet is too close to the metal plate
    B. the venturi gate is stuck open
    C. the air-mix is pushed in
    D. all of the above
    E. A and B only

12-16. The pressure generated during exhalation with a fixed orifice device during PEP therapy will be directly influenced by:
    A. the size of the orifice
    B. the flow rate of gas during exhalation
    C. the patient's respiratory rate
    D. all of the above
    E. A and B only

12-17. The goal of PEP therapy is to
    A. prevent or reverse atelectasis
    B. help in the removal of secretions
    C. cause smooth muscle in the airway to relax
    D. all of the above
    E. A and B only

12-18. Which of the following are true concerning the FIO_2 delivered by the Bird Mark 7, set on air-mix, when powered by 100% oxygen?
    A. the higher the pressure, the higher the FIO_2
    B. the higher the pressure, the more entrainment will occur
    C. long inspiratory times may result in an FIO_2 of less than 30% oxygen
    D. all of the above
    E. A and B only

12-19. An IPPB machine will not cycle off even with the mouth piece occluded. This could be due to which of the following?
   A. a hole in the tubing
   B. a leak at the nebulizer assembly
   C. a leak through the exhalation valve
   D. all of the above
   E. A and B only

13

Classification of Mechanical Ventilators

INTRODUCTION

Knowing the classification scheme for a particular mechanical ventilator does not mean that a respiratory care practitioner (RCP) can operate the machine properly. However, knowledge of ventilator classification contributes to an understanding of machine operation and allows the RCP to use it more appropriately and safely. Chapter 13 discusses the mechanical ventilator classification system, ventilator alarms, volume loss due to compression, and auto-PEEP.

VOLUME LOSS DUE TO COMPRESSION

When patients are being mechanically ventilated, some of the set volume is never delivered to the patient's airway. During inspiration, when the system is pressurized, gas is compressed in the circuit. This compressed gas accounts for what is known as "volume loss due to compression." This volume loss (V_L) robs the patient of alveolar ventilation, and delivered minute ventilation will need to be increased to compensate. (Remember that required minute ventilation is usually documented by ABG analysis.) Several factors affect the amount of volume loss. These include length and volume of the tubing and humidifier system, tubing compliance, and system pressure.

Calculation of Volume Loss

First Step

Calculation of volume loss due to compression should involve a two-step procedure. The first step involves the calculation of the compression factor. This is accomplished by one of two methods. The first method begins with the ventilator and tubing completely assembled, and the patient connection capped. Set a volume on the ventilator of 100–200 mL. Set the pressure limit at its maximum. Adjust the flow rate to a very low value and cycle the ventilator. The machine will volume cycle. Observe the peak inspiratory pressure (PIP) for the delivered volume.

The second method also begins with the ventilator and tubing completely assembled, and the patient connection capped. Set a desired pressure limit at 40–80 cm H_2O. Set the V_t at 500 mL. Adjust the flow rate to a very low value, and cycle the ventilator. The machine will pressure cycle. Observe the delivered volume at the set pressure limit.

Using either method, the compression factor (C_{pc}) is now determined by using the following formula:

$$C_{pc} = \text{delivered } V_t/(PIP - EEP)$$

where

C_{pc} is the compression factor or the compliance of the patient circuit at a given pressure
V_t is the volume used to pressurize the circuit
PIP is peak inspiratory pressure
EEP is the end expiratory or baseline pressure

Example

A 150-mL volume is compressed into a capped circuit at a pressure of 50 cm H_2O. No PEEP is present. The C_{pc} is calculated by dividing 150 mL/50 cm H_2O, equaling 3 mL/cm H_2O. The C_{pc} is the number of milliliters of gas that will be trapped in the circuit for every 1 cm H_2O pressure applied to the system. The C_{pc} will typically fall between 1.5 and 3 mL/cm H_2O for adult circuits, but will vary from circuit to circuit and at different system pressures.

Second Step

The second step in determining the actual volume loss (V_L) is to multiply the compression factor times the actual system pressure during patient ventilation using the following formula:

$$C_{pc} \times \text{ventilating pressure} = V_L$$

Example

A patient is being ventilated and the PIP is 40 cm H_2O. The circuit C_{pc} is measured at 3 mL/cm H_2O. The V_L is calculated by multiplying $C_{pc} \times PIP$—$3 \times 40 = 120$ mL. If a V_t of 700 mL is delivered from the ventilator, only 580 mL (700 – 120) reaches the patient airway. If the patient has a dead space (V_D) of 180 mL, only 400 mL (580 – 180) comprises alveolar ventilation per breath. (Refer to Chapter 17 for a discussion of V_D.)

Note that some mechanical ventilators now have an option which allows the caregiver to choose a compression factor. This option will instruct the ventilator to deliver extra volume to compensate for the volume loss, and it will not be shown as part of the exhaled volume reading.

Measuring Volume Loss Due to Compression

Volume loss, V_L, due to compression can be measured by measuring exhaled gas at two different sites and calculating the difference. One site is at the exhalation valve. The other site is at the endotracheal tube.

Laboratory Exercise

13-1. Using a ventilator and circuit, determine the compliance of the patient circuit. Repeat this exercise for different circuits and at several pressure levels. Record the results.

13-2. Set up a mechanical ventilator in the AC mode and attach it to a test lung. Deliver a set V_t and measure the volume exiting the exhalation port. Also measure the volume exiting from the test lung. A Wright respirometer or similar device can be used. The difference between the two values is the V_L due to compression. Calculate the V_L due to compression based on the compression factor of the circuit. Compare the measured V_L to the calculated V_L.

AUTO-PEEP

Auto-PEEP is present when there is an EEP greater than the set baseline pressure. Auto-PEEP results when expiratory time (T_E) is too short to allow complete exhalation to baseline volume level. This results in increased trapped gas volume in the patient's lungs. Auto-PEEP is an index of that trapped volume. The amount of volume retained in the lungs by PEEP or auto-PEEP can be calculated if the patient's static compliance (C_{st}) is known by using the following formula:

$$\text{Retained (or trapped) volume} = C_{st} \times \text{PEEP}$$

Example

A patient has a C_{st} of 30 mL/cm H_2O. His PEEP level is +10 cm H_2O. His FRC has been increased by 300 mL by the +10 PEEP—30 mL/cm $H_2O \times 10$ cm H_2O = 300 mL. Following some ventilator parameter changes, the patient is experiencing auto-PEEP at a level of +15 cm H_2O. His compliance is still 30 mL/cm H_2O. His total trapped volume is 450 mL—30 mL/cm $H_2O \times 15$ cm H_2O = 450 mL. The auto-PEEP is causing an extra 150 mL of volume to be trapped in his lung.

Laboratory Exercises

13-3. Using a mechanical ventilator and a test lung, create auto-PEEP. Begin with normal ventilation parameters. Then, by increasing the respiratory frequency or increasing inspiratory time (increase V_t or decrease flow), cause the T_E to become very short. Watch the manometer for the development of auto-PEEP. Be aware that auto-PEEP can occur without showing up on the manometer during dynamic gas flow. Refer to *Respiratory Care Equipment* for proper methods for determining auto-PEEP.

REVIEW QUESTIONS

13-4. The power used to operate a mechanical ventilator is called:
A. input power
B. output power
C. force
D. pressure

13-5. The most common forms of input power are:
A. electric
B. pneumatic
C. mechanical
D. all of the above
E. A and B only

13-6. Electric power input may come from:
A. 100 volts AC (Europe)
B. 110 volts AC (America)
C. rechargeable batteries
D. all of the above
E. A and B only

13-7. Advantages of pneumatic ventilators may include:
A. use during transports
B. use during electrical blackouts
C. use during magnetic resonance imaging
D. all of the above
E. A and B only

13-8. Which of the following types of compressors are used inside ventilators?
I. piston
II. diaphragm
III. bellows
IV. rotating vane
A. I and II only
B. III and IV only
C. I, III, and IV only
D. I, II, III, and IV

13-9. Which of the following are true regarding an output control valve?
A. it regulates flow to the patient
B. it may be a simple on/off valve
C. it may shape the waveform of flow delivered to the patient
D. all of the above
E. A and B only

13-10. During mechanical ventilation, which of the following must be measured relative to their baseline value?
A. pressure
B. volume
C. flow
D. all of the above
E. A and B only

13-11. In considering measurements made during mechanical ventilation, which of the following are correct?
   A. pressure should be measured as the change in pressure above PEEP
   B. volume should be measured as the change in volume above FRC
   C. flow should be measured relative to flow at end inspiration
   D. all of the above
   E. A and B only

13-12. A patient's breath is assisted by the ventilator:
   A. only if it is a spontaneous breath
   B. only if it is a mandatory breath
   C. only if the ventilator is in the A/C mode
   D. any time the pressure rises above baseline during inspiration

13-13. During pressure controlled ventilation, the independent variable is:
   A. pressure
   B. volume
   C. flow

13-14. During flow controlled ventilation, the shape of the pressure waveform depends on:
   A. the flow waveform
   B. the patient's airway resistance
   C. the patient's lung/thorax compliance
   D. all of the above
   E. A and B only

13-15. When using pressure, volume, and flow, a ventilator can directly control how many of these variables at a time?
   A. one
   B. two
   C. three

13-16. A control circuit may be which of the following types?
   I. mechanical
   II. pneumatic
   III. fluidic
   IV. electric
   V. electronic
   A. I and II only
   B. II and V only
   C. I, II, and III only
   D. I, III, and IV only
   E. I, II, III, IV, and V

13-17. To qualify as a volume controller, a ventilator must do which of the following?
   A. measure volume
   B. use the volume signal to control the volume waveform
   C. maintain a consistent volume waveform in the face of a varying load
   D. all of the above
   E. A and B only

13-18. When considering one respiratory cycle, phase variables refer to:
    I. pressure
    II. volume
    III. flow
    IV. time
A. I and III
B. II and IV
C. IV only
D. I, II, III, and IV

13-19. In an apneic patient, the most common inspiratory trigger is:
A. pressure
B. volume
C. flow
D. time

13-20. The variable used to end inspiratory time is the:
A. trigger
B. cycle variable
C. limit variable
D. baseline variable

13-21. Instead of inspiration being volume cycled, many third-generation mechanical ventilators are actually:
A. pressure cycled
B. flow cycled
C. time cycled
D. patient cycled

13-22. Which of the following constitutes a spontaneous breath?
    I. patient initiated, patient terminated
    II. patient initiated, ventilator terminated
    III. ventilator initiated, patient terminated
    IV. ventilator initiated, ventilator terminated
A. I only
B. I and II only
C. I, II, and III only
D. I, II, III, and IV

13-23. Which of the following modes are assisted, spontaneous breaths?
A. SIMV
B. pressure support
C. A/C
D. all of the above
E. A and B only

13-24. Another name for accelerating or decelerating flow waveforms is:
A. sinusoidal
B. rectangular
C. ramp
D. exponential

13-25. Given a V_t of 600 mL, a compression factor of 3 mL/cm H_2O, and a PIP of 45 cm H_2O, calculate volume loss due to compression.
A. 15 mL
B. 135 mL
C. 180 mL
D. 200 mL

13-26. Given a V_t of 600 mL, a patient compliance of 60 mL/cm H_2O, and an auto-PEEP of +12 cm H_2O, calculate the amount of air trapped in the patients lungs.
A. 50 mL
B. 72 mL
C. 500 mL
D. 720 mL

13-27. Auto-PEEP results when:
A. T_I is too long
B. T_I is too short
C. T_E is too long
D. T_E is too short

13-28. Volume loss due to compression will result in:
A. decreased volume output by the ventilator
B. decreased alveolar ventilation
C. decreased dead space
D. all of the above
E. A and B only

14

Mechanical Ventilators

INTRODUCTION

Chapter 14 discusses many of the adult and infant ventilators currently in use in hospitals for short- and long-term care. Owing to the number of ventilators on the market, the following laboratory exercises are not ventilator specific, but rather generic in their application.

ADULT VENTILATORS

To understand how a mechanical ventilator operates, one must become familiar with it. This can only be accomplished by reading the literature (operation manual) and by having hands-on experience with the machine. Although ventilators which incorporate pistons, bellows, demand valves, etc. may differ in their operation, the following exercises will help to increase awareness of how ventilators function.

Laboratory Exercises

For each of the following exercises, select a mechanical ventilator, assemble and connect the appropriate circuit, and attach a test lung to the patient connector.

14-1.   Examine the dials, touch pads, etc., and become familiar with their operation. Turn the ventilator on, and adjust the settings for a normal routine patient situation with normal resistance and compliance. Settings are: AC, volume cycled, frequency of 12/min, V_t of 700 mL, (V_E of 8.4 L) FIO_2 of 40%, PEEP of +3 cm H_2O, sensitivity of –2 cm H_2O, flow rate (FR) of 40 L/min, and a pressure limit of 50 cm H_2O. Set other parameters and alarm limits as appropriate. Document the actual exhaled volume and peak inspiratory pressure (PIP) required to deliver the volume. Create a high pressure condition and check for proper alarm and termination of breath. Does the ventilator pressure alarm respond to internal machine pressure or proximal system (patient) pressure? Repeat this exercise with several mechanical ventilators.

14-2.   Actively generating negative pressure by manipulation of the test lung or by breathing on the circuit, test each of the following modes of ventilation: control, AC, IMV/SIMV, pressure support, and pressure control. Be sure to use low pressures and a clean circuit to prevent lung injury or infection if personally breathing on the circuit. Perform this exercise using different ventilators and at different sensitivity settings.

14-3. Select a mechanical ventilator with digital readouts for inspiratory time (T_i), PIP, inspiratory to expiratory ratio (I : E), etc., or obtain an in-line monitor which can measure these parameters. Also obtain a test lung with adjustable resistance and compliance settings. Set up a normal patient situation in the volume-cycled mode with normal resistance (R), compliance (C), and ventilator settings. Document each of the settings: C, R, FR, flow pattern (FP), and V_t. Also document each of the resultants: T_i, PIP, and I : E. After recording each of these, start by making one change at a time and document the effect of that change. Evaluate the effects caused by these changes.

Parameter Change		Resultants	
increase R	T_i _____	PIP _____	I : E _____
decrease R	T_i _____	PIP _____	I : E _____
increase C	T_i _____	PIP _____	I : E _____
decrease C	T_i _____	PIP _____	I : E _____
increase FR	T_i _____	PIP _____	I : E _____
decrease FR	T_i _____	PIP _____	I : E _____
change FP	T_i _____	PIP _____	I : E _____
increase V_t	T_i _____	PIP _____	I : E _____
decrease V_t	T_i _____	PIP _____	I : E _____

14-4. Repeat exercise 14-3 with the ventilator in the time-cycled, pressure-limited (pressure control) mode. Set up a normal patient situation with normal resistance (R), compliance (C), and ventilator settings. Document each of the settings: C, R, FR, T_i, and PIP. Also document the resultant V_t. After documenting each of these, start by making one change at a time and document the effect of that change. Evaluate the effect caused by these changes.

Parameter Change	Resultant
increase R	V_t _____
decrease R	V_t _____
increase C	V_t _____
decrease C	V_t _____
increase FR	V_t _____
decrease FR	V_t _____
increase PIP	V_t _____
decrease PIP	V_t _____

14-5. If a graphics package is available on the mechanical ventilator being studied, evaluate the flow–volume and/or pressure–volume curves generated by the parameter changes made in exercises 14-3 and 14-4.

14-6. Set up a "normal" patient on mechanical ventilation. Document the FIO_2 at the patient connector and the delivered V_t. Using appropriate equipment, deliver an in-line aerosol treatment by two methods:
1. the ventilator's built-in nebulizer system if present and
2. a small-volume nebulizer (SVN) powered from an external flowmeter.
Document the change in FIO_2 and V_t for each of these methods. Does the use of the nebulizer affect the sensitivity of the system? Compare the two methods and list some advantages and disadvantages for each.

14-7. Many mechanical ventilators have a sensitivity setting that is compensated to adjust automatically in the presence PEEP. It is said to "track" the PEEP setting. Set up situations to document whether or not sensitivity tracks PEEP in several mechanical ventilators.

INFANT VENTILATORS

Time-Cycled, Pressure-Limited Ventilation

Usually, infant ventilators are time cycled although some are said to have volume-cycling capabilities. Infant ventilation is often carried out by using a pressure limited mode. This means that a preset pressure limit is reached and held as a pressure plateau for the duration of T_i which is time cycled. Depending on the length of T_i, there are several factors that can affect V_t in this mode of ventilation. For a short T_i, when alveolar pressure (P_{alv}) does not equilibrate with system pressure (P_{sys}), the following may all affect V_t: patient airway resistance and lung–thorax compliance (C) (time constants), PIP, and flow rate. For a longer T_i, when P_{alv} equilibrates with P_{sys}, only ΔP and compliance will determine V_t. ΔP represents the pressure difference between PEEP level and PIP. V_t is directly proportional to both compliance and ΔP. When using this method of ventilation ($P_{alv} = P_{sys}$), volume loss due to compression does not "rob" the patient of volume, or change the actual patient V_t. The actual patient V_t can be measured by using a pneumotachometer placed in the dead space of the circuit, that is, attached to the endotracheal tube. V_t will vary as compliance changes and V_t cannot be calculated unless the patient's compliance is known. The formula for compliance (C) determination is

$$C = \Delta V/\Delta P$$

where ΔV is V_t and ΔP is (PIP – PEEP).

Rewritten

$$\Delta V = C \times \Delta P$$

Example

An infant on a ventilator has a lung compliance of 2 mL/cm H_2O. His PEEP level is +4 cm H_2O and his PIP is 20 cm H_2O. What V_t is delivered to his lungs?

$$\Delta V = C \times \Delta P$$

$$V_t = C \times (PIP - PEEP)$$

$$V_t = 2 \text{ mL/cm } H_2O \times (20 - 4 \text{ cm } H_2O)$$

$$V_t = 2 \times 16 = 32 \text{ mL}$$

Time-Cycled, Volume Constant Ventilation

Another method of infant ventilation is accomplished by setting a desired flow rate and T_i while not pressure limiting. In this case, the delivered V_t is determined by T_i and FR and can be calculated. However, it will not be the actual volume delivered to the patient. During this method of ventilation, volume loss due to compression does "rob" some of the delivered volume. Following is the formula for calculation of the delivered volume.

$$(FR \times T_i)/60 = V_t$$

where
FR is flow rate in liters per minute
T_i is inspiratory time in seconds
60 is number of seconds per minute
V_t is tidal volume in L (multiply by 1000 to convert to mL)

Example

An infant is being ventilated by an infant ventilator set at a flow of 6 L/min and with a T_i of 0.4 sec. A pressure limit is not being reached. Calculate the delivered V_t.

$$(FR \times T_i)/60 = V_t$$

$$(6 \times 0.4)/60 = V_t$$

$$2.4/60 = V_t$$

$$0.04 \text{ L} = V_t$$

$$0.04 \text{ L} \times 1000 \text{ mL/L} = 40 \text{ mL}$$

Although the typical infant circuit will have a compression factor lower than its adult counterpart, volume loss due to compression can be significant. The actual V_t the patient receives can be much less than the volume delivered by the machine during this method of ventilation. Because a pressure limit is not reached, V_t tends to stay a little more consistent even in the face of compliance changes. Also, compliance changes may be followed since increased compliance will result in a lower PIP. Decreased compliance and other factors will also result in an increased PIP. Regardless of the type of ventilation performed, if a leak occurs around the uncuffed tube, volume will be lost and the actual volume may not be the same as the measured or calculated volumes.

Laboratory Exercises

14-8.   Select an infant mechanical ventilator. Assemble the appropriate circuit, and attach a test lung to the patient connector. Examine the dials, touch pads, etc., and become familiar with their operation. Turn the ventilator on and adjust the settings for a normal routine patient situation with normal resistance and compliance using: IMV, time cycled, frequency of 30/min, T_i of 0.5 sec, FIO_2 of 40%, PEEP of +4 cm H_2O, flow rate (FR) of 8 L/min, and a pressure limit of 20 cm H_2O. Set other parameters and alarm limits as appropriate. Create some situations causing alarm responses. Did the alarms respond appropriately? Repeat this exercise with several mechanical ventilators. Notice that pressure limit adjustment for pressure-limited ventilation is not labeled as "inspiratory pressure level above PEEP" as it is in adult ventilators. Upper pressure limits will not be automatically adjusted upward or downward as PEEP levels are changed as they are on adult ventilators. They must be manually adjusted if desired.

REVIEW QUESTIONS

14-9.   After changing the circuit on a mechanical ventilator, the RCP notes that the volume is registering 300 mL less than before and that the peak pressure is half of what it was. Which of the following could be the source of the problem?
   I.   the circuit has a hole in the tubing
   II.   the humidifier is not assembled tightly and a leak is occurring
   III.   the medication nebulizer is not connected tightly and leaks
   A.   I only
   B.   III only
   C.   I and II only
   D.   I, II, and III

14-10.   An infant is being ventilated with a time-cycled, pressure-limited ventilator. He has a peak pressure of 26 cm H_2O and a mean airway pressure of 12 cm H_2O. The RCP shortens the inspiratory time. Which of the following responses would now be expected?
   A.   decreased expiratory phase
   B.   increased peak pressure
   C.   increased tidal volume
   D.   decreased mean airway pressure

14-11.   An RCP is called to the intensive care unit to check an adult patient who is being mechanically ventilated. No exhaled volume is being recorded and the pressure alarm is sounding on each inspiration. The first action should be to:
   A.   call the supervisor
   B.   increase the pressure limit setting
   C.   increase the tidal volume setting
   D.   manually ventilate the patient

14-12. An adult patient is receiving ventilatory support with volume-cycled ventilation with the following settings. Mode: AC; FIO_2: 0.40; V_t: 800 mL; frequency: 12/min. The RCP hears the low volume alarm and observes that the system pressure only reaches 7 cm H_2O during the inspiratory phase. Which of the following should be done?
   A.   reconnect the exhalation valve line
   B.   increase the pressure limit
   C.   straighten the kink in the inspiratory line
   D.   empty the condensate from the circuit
   E.   switch to the control mode of ventilation

14-13. A neonate is receiving pressure-limited mechanical ventilation. The physician requests an increase in mean airway pressure. Which of the following could be recommended?
             I.   increase the inspiratory time
            II.   increase the pressure limit
           III.   increase the expiratory time
   A.   I only
   B.   I and II only
   C.   II and III only
   D.   I, II, and III

14-14. While a patient is being ventilated with a Bennett MA-1 ventilator, the spirometer rises during the inspiratory phase. The most likely cause of this rise is which of the following?
   A.   the exhalation valve is leaking
   B.   the spirometer is leaking
   C.   the cuff of the endotracheal tube is leaking
   D.   the inspiratory flow is too high

14-15. While checking a ventilator that has a heated humidifier, it is noted that there is very little water in the tubing and it does not need to be drained. The most likely explanation is that the :
   A.   ventilator rate is set very low
   B.   heating element is not functioning
   C.   flow is set too low
   D.   room temperature is lower than normal

14-16. If the I : E ratio light on a ventilator (set to illuminate at a 1 : 1 ratio) is illuminating on each breath, which of the following controls could be adjusted to eliminate the light?
             I.   volume
            II.   respiratory rate
           III.   sensitivity
            IV.   inspiratory flow
   A.   I and II only
   B.   II and III only
   C.   IV only
   D.   I, II, and IV only

14-17. A breathing circuit's compression factor is determined by cycling a known volume into an occluded circuit and dividing it by:
   A. peak inspiratory pressure plus baseline pressure
   B. peak inspiratory pressure minus baseline pressure
   C. baseline pressure
   D. end inspiratory pause pressure plus baseline pressure

14-18. Given the following data for an infant ventilator, calculate its tidal volume?
   $T_i = 0.5$ sec, $T_e = 1$ sec,   flow rate = 7 L/min,   pressure limit not reached
   A. 1.6 mL
   B. 5.8 mL
   C. 16 mL
   D. 58 mL
   E. 116 mL

14-19. If the sensitivity control on a ventilator is PEEP-compensated, then:
   A. the greater the PEEP value, the less the sensitivity
   B. PEEP should be applied only in the AC mode
   C. PEEP in the system is dependent on the sensitivity control
   D. PEEP can be applied without altering the inspiratory effort required to trigger the ventilator

14-20. Given the following information, calculate the V_t. $T_i = 0.25$ sec, $T_e = 0.4$ sec, FR = 6 L/min, and a pressure limit is not reached.
   A. 5 mL
   B. 15 mL
   C. 25 mL
   D. 40 mL

14-21. During infant pressure-limited ventilation, V_t is measured at 22 mL, PEEP is +4 cm H_2O, and PIP is 16 cm H_2O. Calculate compliance.
   A. 1.4 mL/cm H_2O
   B. 1.8 mL/cm H_2O
   C. 3.2 mL/cm H_2O
   D. 5.5 mL/cm H_2O

14-22. An infant's compliance, while on pressure-limited mechanical ventilation, is measured to be 1 mL/cm H_2O, PIP is 28 cm H_2O, and PEEP is +6 cm H_2O. Calculate the delivered V_t.
   A. 17 mL
   B. 22 mL
   C. 28 mL
   D. 34 mL

14-23. During pressure-limited ventilation on an infant, the PIP is increased with no other changes. How will this affect the V_t?
   A. increase V_t
   B. decrease V_t
   C. no change in V_t

14-24. During pressure-limited ventilation on an infant, the PEEP level is increased with no other changes. How will this affect V_t?
   A. increase V_t
   B. decrease V_t
   C. no change in V_t

14-25. During time-cycled infant ventilation, when a pressure limit is not reached, decreasing the T_i will have what effect on V_t?
   A. increase V_t
   B. decrease V_t
   C. no change in V_t

14-26. During adult volume-cycled ventilation, increasing the flow rate will result in which of the following?
   A. decreased PIP
   B. decreased T_i
   C. increased V_t
   D. all of the above
   E. A and B only

14-27. During adult volume-cycled ventilation, decreasing the V_t will result in which of the following?
   A. decrease T_i
   B. decrease PIP
   C. increase airway resistance
   D. all of the above
   E. A and B only

14-28. Delivery of an aerosol treatment with a SVN powered by a wall flowmeter will result in which of the following?
   A. decreased sensitivity
   B. increased PIP
   C. increased V_t
   D. all of the above
   E. A and B only

15

Transport Ventilators

INTRODUCTION

Transport of mechanically ventilated patients in the hospital environment, or outside it, creates a unique set of conditions for the health care team involved. Mechanical ventilators provide an alternative to manual bag–valve ventilation for these patients. Chapter 15 describes the desired characteristics of transport ventilators and provides an in-depth discussion of many of the models available for use. Because of the many transport ventilators on the market, the following exercise is generic in nature.

Laboratory Exercise

Hands-on experience is the best way to gain an understanding of ventilator function. For the following exercises, select a transport ventilator, assemble and attach the appropriate circuit, and place a test lung on the patient connector.

15-1.   Examine the knobs, touch pads, etc., on the ventilator and become familiar with their operation. Plug the ventilator into a pressurized gas source, turn the ventilator on, and adjust the settings for a normal routine patient situation.
1. Determine the modes of ventilation available, and select the appropriate one.
2. Set an appropriate respiratory rate.
3. Set the ventilator to deliver a volume of 700 mL. This is often accomplished by setting an inspiratory time and a flow rate.
4. If applicable, adjust the FIO_2. Many transport ventilators deliver the FIO_2 of the source gas (100% oxygen), and it is not adjustable. Analyze the FIO_2.
5. Add PEEP to the system. Is this accomplished by the ventilator or must an external PEEP attachment be used?
6. Adjust sensitivity to –2 cm H_2O. If set prior to the addition of PEEP it may need to be readjusted. Check to see if sensitivity adjusts automatically for PEEP.
7. Adjust high and low pressure limits and other alarm settings as appropriate. Which alarms are present on the machine?
8. Using a volume monitor, measure the volume delivered to the test lung.
9. Create several alarm conditions, and document appropriate alarm response.
10. Repeat this exercise with different settings and with several transport ventilators.

15-2.   In addition to the mechanical ventilator, list other equipment needed during a patient transport.

REVIEW QUESTIONS

15-3.   Which of the following are desirable characteristics for transport ventilators?
   A.   compact
   B.   lightweight
   C.   durable
   D.   all of the above
   E.   A and B only

15-4.   Which of the following are correct for pre-hospital electronic transport ventilators?
   A.   they require two perishable power sources
   B.   they offer more precise control of variables
   C.   they have been preferred to their pneumatically powered counterparts
   D.   all of the above
   E.   A and B only

15-5.   Which of the following are correct for pneumatically powered transport ventilators?
   A.   rate and V_t may change if operated at other than 50 psi where calibrated
   B.   they generally do not consume gas to operate
   C.   they are not adequate for in-hospital patient transport
   D.   all of the above
   E.   A and B only

15-6.   Pre-hospital transport ventilators should be cycled by which of the following?
   A.   time
   B.   flow
   C.   pressure
   D.   all of the above
   E.   A and B only

15-7.   Neonates should be ventilated with which of the following FIO_2s during transport?
   A.   100% O_2
   B.   21% O_2
   C.   variable FIO_2 by using a blender

15-8.   For a transport ventilator, if T_i is set at 1.25 sec and flow rate is set at 600 mL/sec, determine V_t.
   A.   450 mL
   B.   480 mL
   C.   600 mL
   D.   750 mL

15-9. A transport ventilator is being used to ventilate an apneic patient. Flow is set at 60 L/min, T_i at 1 sec, frequency at 12/min, and 100% O_2 is being used. The ventilator also consumes a flow of 10 L/min for its operation. A full E-cylinder will supply oxygen for a maximum of how many minutes?
A.   8 min
B.   28 min
C.   51 min
D.   62 min

15-10. When compared to transports with a mechanical ventilator, the use of manual ventilation with a self-inflating bag during transport can result in which of the following?
A. hyperventilation
B. respiratory acidosis
C. hypertension
D. bradycardia

15-11. For a transport ventilator, if T_i is set at 0.8 sec, flow rate at 50 L/min, and frequency at 14/min, determine V_E.
A.   4.8 L
B.   9.3 L
C.   13.4 L
D.   18.5 L

15-12. For a transport ventilator, if T_i is set at 1.0 sec and flow rate at 800 mL/sec, determine V_t.
A.   600 mL
B.   800 mL
C.   1000 mL
D.   1200 mL

16

Home Mechanical Ventilation Equipment

INTRODUCTION

As change continues to overshadow the health care industry, home care will increasingly become a viable option for patients. In the past, many remained hospitalized for much longer, if not indefinitely. Mechanical ventilation of patients is now included in an array of home therapies. Much of the equipment used to perform mechanical ventilation at home is discussed in Chapter 16.

Laboratory Exercise

Many respiratory care students may not have easy access to mechanical ventilators used in the home setting. If it is possible to acquire one or more models, the following exercise can be conducted.

16-1.
1. Select a home care ventilator, assemble and attach the circuit, and place a test lung on the patient connector.
2. Examine the knobs and touch pads on the ventilator and become familiar with their function.
3. Turn the ventilator on and adjust the settings for a routine patient situation.
4. Evaluate the alarm package available on the machine. Set up various alarm conditions, and document the appropriate alarm response.
5. Deliver supplemental oxygen to the system. Using the manufacturer's FIO_2 calculation method, calculate and then analyze the delivered FIO_2.
6. Add PEEP to the system. Determine how this affects sensitivity and the imposed work of breathing.
7. Repeat this exercise with another home care ventilator.

REVIEW QUESTIONS

16-2. Which of the following are correct concerning the rocking bed?
   A. it works well for patients with COPD
   B. it is used primarily for daytime ventilatory assistance
   C. breath rate is fixed
   D. all of the above
   E. A and B only

16-3. Which of the following are correct concerning the pneumobelt?
   A. an inflatable pressurized bladder actively aids with inspiration
   B. proper use increases FRC
   C. the device's effectiveness changes as patient position changes
   D. all of the above
   E. A and B only

16-4. Which of the following are correct concerning negative pressure chambers?
   A. leaks are a common problem
   B. the Iron Lung is an example of a full body chamber
   C. the cuirass is placed over the patient's chest and abdomen
   D. all of the above
   E. A and B only

16-5. Which of the following are correct concerning negative pressure generators?
   A. the Iron Lung is the standard for negative ventilation
   B. patient acceptance is improved when I : E ratio is variable and assisted ventilation is an option
   C. some devices provide a positive pressure phase to aid in exhalation
   D. all of the above
   E. A and B only

16-6. Which of the following are correct concerning home care positive pressure ventilators?
   A. reliability is of great importance
   B. in general, the more alarms the better
   C. SIMV is an absolute requirement
   D. all of the above
   E. A and B only

16-7. Which of the following would describe the ideal positive pressure ventilator for home care patients?
   A. simple
   B. straightforward
   C. user-friendly
   D. all of the above
   E. A and B only

16-8. Which of the following are correct concerning BiPAP devices?
   A. they are generally designed for noninvasive use
   B. they allow two pressure levels to be set (inspiration and expiration)
   C. most units are designed for use with patients who can sustain spontaneous breathing

    D.   all of the above

    E.   A and B only

16-9.   Which of the following are correct concerning oxygen delivery by mechanical ventilators used in the home?

    A.   most provide a precise control of oxygen greater than 21%

    B.   the F_{IO_2} may be increased in all units with proper adapters

    C.   ventilatory rate and V_t have no affect on delivered F_{IO_2}

    D.   all of the above

    E.   A and B only

16-10. Which of the following are correct concerning imposed work of breathing (WOB) for ventilators used at home?

    A.   imposed WOB is increased in the SIMV mode

    B.   a bubble-through humidifier can more than double the WOB

    C.   it is recommended that only the AC mode be used on home care patients to help reduce the WOB

    D.   all of the above

    E.   A and B only

16-11. Which of the following are correct concerning PEEP and home care ventilators?

    A.   PEEP can be applied to any home care ventilator

    B.   sensitivity tracks PEEP on home care ventilators

    C.   imposed WOB does not increase with the use of PEEP

    D.   all of the above

    E.   A and B only

16-12. Appliances for delivery of noninvasive positive pressure ventilation may include:

    A.   nasal masks

    B.   mouthpieces

    C.   nasal pillows

    D.   all of the above

    E.   A and B only

17

High Frequency Ventilators

INTRODUCTION

Compared with conventional mechanical ventilation, high frequency ventilation (HFV) is a mode of therapy with which many RCPs have had minimal clinical experience. The lack of knowledge surrounding many of the concepts involved in HFV results in hesitancy in initiating this form of therapy. Likewise, until clinical trials demonstrate clear benefits of the different HFV modalities, their use will probably remain in the shadows.

DEAD SPACE

Dead space (V_D) can be simply defined as ventilation without gas exchange. The conducting airways (anatomic dead space) are responsible for most of *normal* V_D. Another type of V_D is *alveolar* V_D and is found in alveoli that are ventilated but not perfused with blood. Alveolar V_D will increase in some disease states such as pulmonary embolization. The combination of anatomic and alveolar V_D makes up physiologic V_D. An approximation of normal V_D is 1 mL/lb ideal body weight. *Mechanical* V_D can be defined as rebreathed gas and is present in the tubing of patient connectors through which patients both inhale and exhale. Most commonly, this occurs during mechanical ventilation. If all other parameters remain constant, increasing mechanical dead space will result in an increased $PaCO_2$.

The concept of V_D is important in the discussion of HFV and may have posed a road block to the development of HFV. For a long time, it has been suggested that a V_t greater than V_D is needed to supply fresh air to the alveoli. This is the alveolar ventilation or bulk gas flow theory for gas transport. This theory suggests that if a V_t equal to or less than an individual's V_D is delivered for a period of time, the alveoli will not receive fresh gas. In turn, this would result in an increase in $PaCO_2$ and a decrease in PaO_2. HFV has demonstrated that small volumes of gas can maintain appropriate alveolar ventilation. This finding has led to and helped to substantiate other theories of gas transport that are presented in *Respiratory Care Equipment*.

Laboratory Exercise

If it is possible to acquire one or more types of high frequency ventilators, the following exercise can be performed.

17-1. 1. Select a high frequency ventilator, assemble and attach the circuit, and place a test lung on the connector.
2. Examine the knobs and touch pads on the ventilator and become familiar with their function.
3. Turn the ventilator on and adjust the settings for a routine patient.
4. Make changes in frequency, T_i, driving pressure, respiratory impedance, bias flow, etc., and document the effects on V_t and other parameters.
5. Evaluate the alarm package available on the machine. Set up various alarm conditions and document the appropriate alarm response.

REVIEW QUESTIONS

17-2. Which of the following are correct concerning HFPPV?
  A. a major advantage has been its use in the operating room
  B. most HFV of neonates is a form of HFPPV
  C. the use of HFPPV in acute respiratory failure is well documented
  D. all of the above
  E. A and B only

17-3. Which of the following are correct concerning HFJV?
  A. jet mixing is incorporated into this mode of therapy
  B. rates greater than 200 cpm appear to be optimum for adults
  C. there is little chance of barotrauma even with inverse I : E ratios
  D. all of the above
  E. A and B only

17-4. During HFJV, V_t can be affected by which of the following?
  A. driving pressure
  B. catheter size
  C. % T_i
  D. all of the above
  E. A and B only

17-5. Which of the following are correct concerning HFJV?
  A. changes in patient compliance and resistance will result in inconsistent V_ts
  B. unacceptable levels of inadvertent PEEP may develop when % T_i is at 0.5% or greater
  C. catheter position near the carina appears to be the best for entrainment
  D. all of the above
  E. A and B only

17-6. FDA-approved indications for HFJV include use for which of the following?
  A. bronchopleural fistulae
  B. pulmonary interstitial emphysema
  C. bronchoscopy
  D. all of the above
  E. A and B only

17-7. Which of the following are correct concerning HFO?
A. clinical trials have demonstrated the superiority of HFO in infants with RDS
B. bias flow improves humidification but does not affect V_t
C. HFO results in both active inspiration and expiration
D. all of the above
E. A and B only

17-8. Which of the following are correct concerning HFPV?
A. at low rates, CO_2 elimination is improved
B. at high rates, oxygenation is improved
C. a demand valve allows for spontaneous breathing
D. all of the above
E. A and B only

17-9. Gas transport during HFV may occur by which of the following means?
A. collateral ventilation
B. facilitated diffusion
C. pendelluft
D. all of the above
E. A and B only

17-10. Collateral ventilation may occur through which of the following?
A. pores of Kohn
B. canals of Lambert
C. foramen of Bachdalek
D. all of the above
E. A and B only

17-11. Gas transport via bulk gas flow is associated with which of the following?
A. spontaneous ventilation
B. conventional mechanical ventilation
C. HFPPV
D. all of the above
E. A and B only

17-12. Which of the following would be an estimate of an individual's V_D if he is 6 feet tall and weighs 170 lb?
A. 80 mL
B. 130 mL
C. 170 mL
D. 240 mL

18

Spontaneous Breathing Systems: IMV and CPAP

INTRODUCTION

Both intermittent mandatory ventilation (IMV) and continuous positive airway pressure (CPAP) gained popularity in the early 1970s. Since then, some of the equipment used to administer these modes of therapy have undergone a great deal of change. *Respiratory Care Equipment* describes the three basic types of IMV systems and their methods of operation. Spontaneous positive end expiratory pressure (sPEEP) and CPAP are also discussed. The current-generation ventilators have built-in SIMV and CPAP/PEEP modalities, which need no extra tubing or adapters for operation. The purpose of Chapter 18 is not to elaborate on these built-in systems (discussed in Chapter 14) but to describe the free-standing systems and those that can be adapted to mechanical ventilators that do not have a built-in system.

IMV, SIMV, AND CPAP

IMV/SIMV

In its simplest form, IMV means that the mechanical ventilator will deliver a preset rate and volume (in the volume-cycled mode) to the patient. If the patient is breathing faster than the preset rate, the patient's spontaneous breaths will be unassisted. By decreasing the mechanical rate on the ventilator, IMV allows the patient to take over progressively more of the work of breathing while the ventilator does less. Some of the new generation ventilators are a little more complicated in that they offer other options. IMV can take place in modes other than the volume-cycled mode, and pressure support (PS) can assist the normally unassisted breaths. A problem encountered with IMV is that the ventilator would cycle at a predetermined time regardless of what the patient was doing, inhaling or exhaling. This problem was overcome by replacing IMV with SIMV, a mode in which ventilator-assisted breaths are synchronized with the patient's respiratory cycle.

CPAP/PEEP

CPAP and PEEP, although used to achieve the same goals, are technically different. This has been addressed in the accompanying *Respiratory Care Equipment*. There can be confusion as to the appropriate use of each term. In general, when the CPAP designation is used, the implication is that the patient is breathing spontaneously without any ventilator assistance. On the other hand, the PEEP designation often implies that mechanically assisted breaths are being used simultaneously. The problem that results in confusion is that this general rule does not always apply. Furthermore, there are some practitioners who may disagree with it. Make sure the patient's respiratory support status is well communicated to all those involved with the care.

Laboratory Exercises

18-1.   1. Set up an open-circuit/parallel-flow IMV circuit. Use Figure 18-2 in *Respiratory Care Equipment* as a guide. These systems have commonly been called H-valve IMV systems due to their configuration. Because these systems are an "extra" on the ventilator circuit, they do not allow synchrony with the patient's respiratory cycle.
   2. Breathe through the system, noting the amount of resistance encountered. Make sure the sensitivity on the ventilator is decreased so that the inspiratory efforts do not cycle the ventilator into inspiration but allow the one-way valve to open into the H-valve.
   3. Make sure the FIO_2 in the parallel flow circuit is set the same as the FIO_2 on the ventilator. Analyze it.
   4. Add low levels of PEEP to the system. Is there a change in the amount of work of breathing encountered?

18-2.   1. Set up a closed-circuit/continuous-flow IMV circuit. Use Figure 18-3. *Respiratory Care Equipment* as a guide. Include an anti-asphyxia (one-way inlet) valve. This is not shown in the figure. Because these systems are an "extra" on the ventilator circuit, they do not allow synchrony with the patient's respiratory cycle.
   2. Breathe through the system, noting the amount of resistance encountered. Vary the flow rate and subjectively document change in resistance to breathing. Make sure the sensitivity on the ventilator is decreased so that the inspiratory efforts do not cycle the ventilator into inspiration.
   3. Make sure the FIO_2 in the continuous flow circuit is set the same as the FIO_2 on the ventilator. Analyze it.
   4. Add low levels of PEEP to the system. Is there a change in the amount of work of breathing encountered?

18-3.   Compare the previous types of IMV systems to one or more SIMV systems that are built into a ventilator. Is the work of breathing greater or less than with the previous systems?

18-4.   Set up an sPEEP system as illustrated in Figure 18-6 of *Respiratory Care Equipment*. Breathe through the system at various low levels of sPEEP. Note the change in the work of breathing.

18-5. Set up a CPAP system as illustrated in Figure 18-9 of *Respiratory Care Equipment*. Breathe through the system at various low levels of CPAP. Note the change in the work of breathing.

18-6. If available, set up another type of CPAP system using a pneumatic or electronic device. How does the work of breathing compare to those already tested?

REVIEW QUESTIONS

18-7. IMV was originally used for which of the following?
A. ventilatory support for post-op patients
B. ventilatory support for infants with HMD
C. ventilatory support for COPD patients
D. ventilatory support for patients with bronchopulmonary fistulas

18-8. Which of the following mechanisms are employed to supply IMV?
A. demand valve systems
B. open-circuit systems
C. closed-circuit systems
D. all of the above
E. A and B only

18-9. With parallel-flow IMV, addition of PEEP to the ventilator system will result in which of the following?
A. an increased inspiratory force required by the patient
B. increased work of breathing
C. increased chance of patient fatigue
D. all of the above
E. A and B only

18-10. The flow necessary for a continuous-flow IMV system can be set appropriately by which of the following methods?
A. Assessing minimal pressure deflections
B. subjective assessment of work of breathing
C. setting flow two times minute ventilation
D. all of the above
E. A and B only

18-11. Placing the valve assembly of a continuous-flow IMV system proximal to the humidifier on the ventilator will result in which of the following?
A. only part of the gas delivered to the patient being humidified
B. possible increased work of breathing if the flow is not high enough
C. inability to deliver PEEP
D. all of the above
E. A and B only

18-12. Pressure monitoring should take place at which of the following sites during continuous-flow IMV ventilation?
A. inside the ventilator (machine pressure)

    B.   just proximal to the humidifier
    C.   just distal to the humidifier
    D.   at the patient's airway (proximal airway pressure)

18-13. Demand valves can be routinely triggered to deliver flow during IMV by which of the following parameters?
    A.   flow
    B.   pressure
    C.   time
    D.   all of the above
    E.   A and B only

18-14. Which of the following are correct when comparing sPEEP to CPAP?
    A.   sPEEP results in a decreased work of breathing when compared to CPAP at the same expiratory pressure
    B.   decreased cardiac output is more likely to occur with sPEEP than CPAP at the same expiratory pressure
    C.   a greater transpulmonary pressure is generated during inspiration with sPEEP than CPAP at the same expiratory pressure
    D.   all of the above
    E.   A and B only

18-15. Which of the following alarms is most important to ensure maintenance of therapy for an adult patient with mask CPAP?
    A.   high F_{IO_2}
    B.   high respiratory rate
    C.   low pressure
    D.   pulse oximetry

18-16. A continuous-flow CPAP system pressure is set at 10 cm H_2O. The manometer decreases to 3 cm H_2O on inspiration but returns to 10 cm H_2O during exhalation. Which of the following is most likely the cause of the problem?
    A.   the flow of gas is too low
    B.   there is a leak in the system
    C.   the CPAP pressure is set too high
    D.   the CPAP valve is too small

18-17. After initiating nasal CPAP therapy on an infant, it is noticed that the system pressure cannot be maintained. Which of the following is most likely the problem?
    A.   a pneumothorax is present
    B.   the exhalation port is blocked
    C.   the prongs are occluded with secretions
    D.   the baby is crying

19

Expiratory Pressure Valves

INTRODUCTION

Inspiratory and expiratory valves are components of many types of equipment used in the practice of respiratory care. From microprocessor-controlled mechanical ventilators to pocket masks for rescue breathing, valves play an important role in the delivery of therapy. Chapter 19 discusses expiratory valves used to regulate end expiratory pressure during either spontaneous or mechanical ventilation. The main types of valves presented are threshold resistors and flow resistors.

THRESHOLD RESISTORS

A true threshold resistor should maintain a constant system pressure even in the face of large flow rate changes. This is accomplished by changing the size of the exhalation port as flow changes. This port becomes larger with increased flows and smaller with lesser flows. In reality, these resistors are variable orifice devices. In clinical practice, a true threshold resistor is difficult to find, although some valves perform much better than others.

FLOW RESISTORS

Use of flow resistors results in system pressure changes as flow rates change. A flow resistor has a fixed orifice. As increased flow attempts to squeeze through the fixed orifice, pressure proximal to the restriction increases. Sometimes the resultant peak pressure fluctuation could be considered excessive. Figure 19-1 on the next page depicts the pressure–flow-rate relationship for both threshold resistors and flow resistors.

Laboratory Exercise

19-1.   Select several types of valves used to create CPAP. Include both flow resistors and threshold resistors. Set up a CPAP assembly for spontaneous breathing. Take one valve at a time, set at a desired pressure level, and measure the pressure change as flow through the valve is increased from 10 to 100 L/min. Document the pressure change. Which valves behave like threshold resistors? Which behave more like a flow resistor?

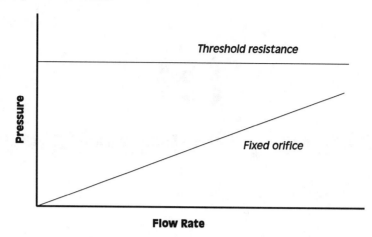

Figure 19-1. Graph illustrating the change in pressure as flow rate changes for both threshold resistors and flow resistors.

REVIEW QUESTIONS

19-2. Which of the following responds more like a flow resistor than a threshold resistor?
A. Siemens servo-controlled "scissor valve"
B. Boehringer weighted-ball valve
C. Emerson water column
D. Vital signs spring loaded disk

19-3. Concerning a flow resistor, which of the following is correct?
A. as flow increases, pressure decreases
B. as flow increases, pressure increases
C. as flow increases, pressure remains constant

19-4. Concerning flow resistors, which of the following is correct at a given flow rate?
A. as orifice size is increased, pressure decreases
B. as orifice size is increased, pressure increases
C. as orifice size is increased, pressure remains constant

19-5. Concerning a threshold resistor, which of the following is correct?
A. as flow increases, pressure decreases
B. as flow increases, pressure increases
C. as flow increases, pressure remains constant

19-6. Increased resistance to expiratory flow may result in which of the following?
A. increased imposed WOB
B. increased peak exhalation pressure
C. decreased venous return
D. all of the above
E. A and B only

19-7. Which of the following is recommended as the valve of choice for CPAP systems?
A. high flow-resistant threshold resistor valves
B. low flow-resistant threshold resistor valves
C. flow resistors

20

Decontamination of Respiratory Care Equipment

INTRODUCTION

Maintaining asepsis is a vital part of all health care practitioners' work. Some reasons for practicing microbial control include: preventing spoilage and decomposition of materials, preventing contamination by or growth of undesired microbes, and preventing transmission of infection and disease. Contaminated equipment can result in nosocomial infections (infections acquired while in the hospital), increased patient morbidity and mortality rates, and increased medical care costs. Actual cleaning and sterilization of equipment may take place in the department of respiratory care or in a central supply area. Many guidelines are now imposed on those who perform these tasks. Respiratory care practitioners are not routinely responsible for the maintenance or repair of the devices used in the sterilization process. Consequently, RCPs should be more concerned with the types of sterilization processes available, their advantages and disadvantages, their practical uses, and the factors affecting the outcomes of these processes.

DECONTAMINATION METHODS

Methods used to help prevent transmission of undesired microbes include hand washing, the use of filters, decontamination processes, and protective equipment—including gloves, masks, and gowns. The common processes used for decontamination of respiratory care equipment are discussed in *Respiratory Care Equipment*. Listed below is a summary of the normal uses, advantages, and disadvantages of these processes.

Soaps and Detergents
Use: hand washing and cleaning debris from equipment. It removes organic material and reduces microbial flora.

Acetic Acid
Use: home care disinfection.
Advantages: simple and cheap.
Disadvantages: not effective against all microbes.
Mode of Action: lowers intracellular pH and inactivates enzymes.

Quaternary Ammonium Compounds or "Quats"

Use: equipment cleaning.
Advantages: quick and easy; noncaustic; relatively nontoxic; no noxious fumes.
Disadvantages: not effective against all microbes.
Mode of Action: membrane lysis and inactivation of cellular enzymes.

Alcohol

Use: skin antiseptic; preparation for arterial and venous punctures; wiping of nonimmersible respiratory equipment.
Advantages: no need to rinse; inexpensive; rapid.
Disadvantages: volatile; damages some plastics and rubber; has limited application.
Mode of Action: denatures proteins and dissolves lipids.

Glutaraldehyde

Use: disinfection/sterilization of hospital equipment.
Advantages: can be used at room temperature; will not harm rubber and plastics with short-term exposure; simple to use; relatively inexpensive; rapid.
Disadvantages: irritating odor; contact dermatitis; may be corrosive to some metals; equipment must be rinsed; equipment cannot be prepackaged; processing room must be well ventilated
Mode of Action: attacks lipoproteins in cell membranes and cytoplasm

Hydrogen-Peroxide-Based Compounds

Use: disinfection/sterilization of hospital equipment.
Advantages: safe with rubber, plastic, and stainless steel; no harsh fumes.
Disadvantages: equipment cannot be prewrapped.
Mode of Action: oxidation.

Dry Heat

Use: sterilization of equipment impermeable to steam (oils and powders) or damaged by moisture (sharp instruments).
Advantages: simple and cheap; no residues.
Disadvantages: equipment cannot be prewrapped; cannot process heat-sensitive items.
Mode of Action: desiccation; alteration of osmotic pressure; coagulation of protein; oxidation.

Boiling Water

Use: disinfection of home care equipment; sanitizing of bedding and dishes.
Advantages: simple and cheap; no residues.
Disadvantages: not effective against all microbes; possible danger for home patients due to presence of the hot water bath.
Mode of Action: coagulation of protein.

Pasteurization

Use: disinfection of hospital equipment.
Advantages: cheap; easy; no residues.
Disadvantages: not effective against all microbes.
Mode of Action: coagulation of protein.

Steam Autoclave

Use: sterilization of non-heat-sensitive materials, instruments, and linens; limited use for respiratory care equipment.

Advantages: very reliable; equipment can be prewrapped; rapid; economical; no toxic residues; equipment available for immediate use.

Disadvantages: cannot be used for heat-sensitive items; may blunt and rustinstruments; cannot be used for materials impervious to steam.

Mode of Action: lysis of cell membranes and coagulation of proteins.

Ethylene Oxide (EtO)

Use: sterilization of heat-sensitive equipment; excellent application for respiratory care equipment.

Advantages: equipment can be prewrapped; reliable; operates at relatively low temperatures

Disadvantages: toxic to human tissues; flammable and explosive; possible presence of toxic residues: EtO gas, Ethylene glycol, and ethylene chlorohydrin; aeration is needed; may crack some plastics with repeated use; is carcinogenic and possibly mutagenic and teratogenic; expensive.

Mode of Action: alkylation; denaturing of protein and nucleic acids.

Filters

Use: to physically remove microbes from gas streams especially during mechanical ventilation. These filters are said to have an efficiency of greater than 99.9% for microbes larger than 0.3 microns. This allows for the filtering out of most microbes except viruses.

Gamma Radiation

Use: commercial use by manufacturers for sterilization of disposable respiratory care equipment

Advantages: can be performed at room temperatures; equipment can be prewrapped; fast and effective; equipment ready for immediate use.

Disadvantages: expensive; dangerous radiation; special equipment is needed

Mode of Action: ionization of water molecules and inactivation of DNA molecules

REVIEW QUESTIONS

20-1. Equipment exposed to EtO must not have free-standing water on it to prevent formation of:
A. ethylene glycol
B. ethylene chlorohydrin
C. ethylene chloride
D. ethylene dioxide

20-2. Boiling water would be most effective in killing microbes when occurring:
A. at an elevation of 10,000 ft
B. at an elevation of 5,000 ft
C. at sea level
D. under 1.2 P_{atm} (hyperbaric conditions)

20-3. Most cases of nosocomial pneumonia are caused by:
A. fungi
B. protozoa
C. viruses
D. bacteria

20-4. The main advantage of EtO over other chemical means of sterilization is that:
A. EtO is less toxic
B. equipment can be prewrapped
C. EtO is very effective at room temperature
D. equipment processed using EtO can be used immediately

20-5. Wrapping materials to avoid with use of EtO processing include:
    I. muslin
    II. nylon film
    III. polyethylene
    IV. polyester
A. I and II only
B. II and III only
C. I and III only
D. II and IV only

20-6. To ensure sterility, a properly cleaned piece of equipment needs to be soaked for how long in a glutaraldehyde solution?
A. 10–20 minutes
B. 1–2 hours
C. 3–10 hours
D. 12 hours

20-7. A piece of equipment, sterilized with glutaraldehyde, may be recontaminated during:
    I. rinsing
    II. drying
    III. packaging
    IV. extended shelf life
A. I and II only
B. II and III only
C. I, III, and IV
D. I, II, III, and IV

20-8. Instructions for cleaning a small volume nebulizer by a patient receiving home respiratory therapy treatments include:
    I. thorough washing
    II. rinsing with water
    III. soaking in a vinegar solution
    IV. passively air dry
A. I and II only
B. I, II, and III only
C. II, III, and IV only
D. I, II, III, and IV

20-9. A pulmonary infection outbreak occurs in a unit containing numerous mechanically ventilated patients. The most likely cause of this is:
A. poor air exchange in the patient's room
B. poor hand-washing techniques by personnel
C. an outbreak of the infection in a neighboring hospital
D. poor compliance with isolation techniques

20-10. Saline containers should not be used more than 24 hours after opening because:
A. minerals will precipitate out of solution
B. chemicals will be drawn out of the plastic jar into the solution
C. bacterial contamination may occur
D. evaporation will cause increased sodium concentration

20-11. Sterilization is best defined as a process that:
A. impedes growth of microbes
B. kills all bacteria
C. kills all microbes except spores
D. kills all microbes including viruses and spores

20-12. Which of the following would most likely result in sterilization?
A. steam autoclave
B. EtO gas
C. pasteurization
D. all of the above
E. A and B only

20-13. Autoclave sterilization is a process incorporating which of the following?
I. steam
II. pressure (above atmospheric)
III. temperatures 25–60°C
IV. a sealed chamber
A. I and II only
B. I, II, and III
C. I, II, and IV
D. I, II, III, and IV

20-14. Autoclaving kills microbes by:
A. direct squeezing of the microbe by pressure
B. coagulation of cellular proteins
C. the process of alkylation
D. all of the above
E. A and B only

20-15. Which of the following are true statements concerning the use of EtO for sterilization?
I. the gas is flammable
II. the gas is toxic to human tissues
III. temperature does not affect the time needed for sterilization
IV. humidity does affect the efficiency of the sterilization process
A. I and II only
B. I and III only
C. I, II, and IV
D. II, III, and IV

20-16. When processing equipment, which of the following will best confirm that sterilization has occurred?
- A. physical indicators used during processing
- B. chemical indicators used during processing
- C. biological indicators used during processing
- D. following the manufacturer's instructions for processing

20-17. Filtration of gases delivered to patients results in:
- A. sterilization of the gas
- B. physical removal of microbes
- C. microbial death by chemical means
- D. all of the above
- E. A and B only

20-18. Which of the following are true concerning use of an autoclave?
- A. it is a very reliable method for sterilization
- B. it utilizes Charles' law
- C. pockets of air in the chamber have little effect on sterilization capabilities
- D. all of the above
- E. A and B only

20-19. Bacterial spores are:
- A. the means by which bacteria reproduce
- B. the means by which bacteria survive harsh environments
- C. easily destroyed
- D. all of the above
- E. A and B only

20-20. A microbe with a rod shape is called a:
- A. coccus
- B. spirochete
- C. virion
- D. bacillus

20-21. Staphylococci are seen under a microscope as:
- A. chain-like structures
- B. rod shaped
- C. grape-like clusters
- D. groups of two

20-22. Which of the following is not a complete living cell?
- A. virus
- B. bacterium
- C. fungus
- D. protozoa

20-23. One of the easiest and most effective means to prevent transmission of infection is to:
- A. wear a lab coat
- B. observe proper isolation technique
- C. sterilize all equipment used in a patient's room
- D. wash hands between patient contact

21

Computers and Respiratory Care Equipment

INTRODUCTION

Chapter 21 covers computers for general use as well their use in respiratory care. As the computer information age continues, respiratory care practitioners can expect their profession to become more computer dependent. Hospitals already use computerized charting to cut down on paperwork and save time. For respiratory care, computer technology is involved in everything from arterial blood gas analysis to mechanical ventilators. Pulmonary function lab personnel rely extensively on computerization when performing diagnostic procedures.

"Expert systems" are now being incorporated into hospitals to help in diagnosis of diseases by using a type of flowchart logic. This application can also be seen in the respiratory care profession, since many therapist-driven protocols can also be handled in this manner.

With the inevitable expanding use of computers in the respiratory care profession, it is worthwhile for respiratory students to take at least a basic computer course during their educational career. The course should provide a solid foundation of computer operation on which future knowledge can be built.

A word of caution concerning "de-skilling" is appropriate. De-skilling occurs when a care provider is trained to do a job only with the help of a computer. Thus the care provider becomes a tool of the computer rather than vice versa. With advanced technology becoming more commonplace in the healthcare environment, it is important that RCPs do not become totally dependent on computers to perform the tasks. Therefore, it is vital that an appropriate clinical knowledge base be acquired. It is also important that all facets of a patient's condition be assessed before allowing important clinical decisions to be made, even by a computer.

REVIEW QUESTIONS

21-1. Which of the following types of computer memory is volatile (that is, easily changed by the operator)?
A. ROM
B. RAM
C. REM
D. all of the above
E. A and B only

21-2. Computers can be classified as which of the following?
A. mainframe
B. personal
C. portable
D. all of the above
E. A and B only

21-3. The CPU of a computer does which of the following?
A. performs arithmetic
B. performs logical decisions
C. stores data
D. all of the above
E. A and B only

21-4. Which of the following is not classified as hardware?
A. the disk drive
B. the monitor
C. the printer
D. the programs on diskettes

21-5. Which device converts analog signals to digital and back again?
A. the modem
B. the central processing unit
C. the CRT
D. the operating system

21-6. Operating system software performs which of the following functions?
A. instructs hardware
B. interfaces with keyboard, monitor, etc.
C. performs statistical analysis
D. all of the above
E. A and B only

21-7. Computers in the blood gas lab may perform or control which of the following functions?
A. storage and reporting of values
B. calibration and cleaning
C. timing and endpoint detection
D. all of the above
E. A and B only

21-8. Computerized blood gas interpretation may involve which of the following?
     I.   determination of acid–base status
     II.   alerting to life-threatening conditions
     III.   detection of electrode failure
     IV.   determination of oxygenation status
     V.   comparison with former data
  A. I and IV only
  B. I, II, and IV only
  C. I, II, III, and IV
  D. I, II, IV, and V

21-9. Microprocessor-controlled ventilators are characterized by which of the following?
  A. operator-selected ventilator modes
  B. operator-selected flow patterns
  C. use of electromechanical valves
  D. all of the above
  E. A and B only

21-10. Which of the following types of monitoring is based on mathematical modeling and rule-based logic?
  A. statistical monitoring
  B. analytical monitoring
  C. integrative monitoring
  D. time and limit monitoring

21-11. Computer-based information systems can perform which of the following?
     I.   increased speed and efficiency of charting
     II.   eliminate charting errors
     III.   improve readability of chart
     IV.   standardize the clinical chart
  A. I and III only
  B. I, II, and III only
  C. I, III, and IV only
  D. I, II, III, and IV

21-12. Which of the following are true concerning third-generation hand-held computers?
     I.   inexpensive and not expandable
     II.   can be interfaced with other computers
     III.   limited memory due to size
     IV.   may have decision-making capabilities
  A. I and III only
  B. II and IV only
  C. II, III, and IV only
  D. I, II, III, and IV

21-13. An intensive care unit computer system should be able to
  A. acquire data
  B. communicate data
  C. function as a decision-making tool
  D. all of the above
  E. A and B only

21-14. The evaluation of high and low blood pressure limits is an example of which of the following types of monitoring?
A. statistical monitoring
B. analytical monitoring
C. integrative monitoring
D. time and limit monitoring

21-15. Common computer functions for a Respiratory Care Department would include which of the following?
A. automatic billing
B. order entry
C. shift report
D. all of the above
E. A and B only

22

Approval and Surveillance of Medical Devices

INTRODUCTION

Information concerning medical device approval and post-market surveillance of medical devices is of interest to manufacturers, researchers, and to practitioners as well. Respiratory care practitioners are extensively involved in the clinical setting and use many types of medical devices when performing therapies. It is important to understand the procedures involved for reporting problems encountered with either equipment or medications. *Respiratory Care Equipment* covers these areas and includes the telephone numbers and examples of report forms used by different reporting programs.

REVIEW QUESTIONS

22-1.   To be defined as a medical device, which of the following criteria must be met?
  A.   it does not achieve its purpose through chemical reaction within or on the body
  B.   it does not depend on being metabolized to achieve its purposes
  C.   it is intended to affect structure or function of the body
  D.   all of the above
  E.   A and B only

22-2.   Which class of medical devices applies only to those that are life supporting or life sustaining?
  A.   general controls
  B.   performance standards
  C.   pre-market approval

22-3.   Which of the following is the minimum regulatory control that the FDA requires for distribution into interstate commerce?
  A.   general controls
  B.   performance standards
  C.   pre-market approval

22-4. PMA applications submitted to the FDA by manufacturers must include which of the following?
      I.   indication for use
      II. device description
      III. all significant unpublished clinical investigations
      IV. experimental study design
      V. data collection and analysis of results
  A. I, II, IV, and V only
  B. I, II, III, and IV only
  C. I, III, and IV only
  D. I, II, III, IV, and V

22-5. Before clinical trials can begin on an unapproved device, the manufacturer must obtain which of the following?
  A. written permission from the FDA
  B. an Investigational Device Exemption (IDE)
  C. a 501(k) submission
  D. all of the above
  E. A and B only

22-6. Which of the following is the voluntary reporting system used to report problems with medical devices? It was conceived in 1974.
  A. Device Problem Reporting Program (PRP)
  B. Mandatory Medical Device Reporting Program (MDR)
  C. MEDWATCH Voluntary Reporting Program

22-7. Most of the reported problems for anesthesia and respiratory care are in the area of:
  A. death
  B. injury
  C. malfunctions

22-8. Some of the factors considered by the FDA to determine whether to issue a notification on a medical device include:
  A. whether notification can eliminate risk
  B. number and traceability of the device
  C. severity of harm presented by the risk of using the device
  D. all of the above
  E. A and B only

22-9. Which of the following is true concerning MEDWATCH?
  A. it is a mandatory reporting program
  B. it is intended for reporting all adverse events
  C. forms can be obtained from the FDA
  D. all of the above
  E. A and B only

22-10. In response to the incidence of disconnection of breathing circuits, the ECRI has recommended which of the following?
- A. in-service education
- B. use of disconnect alarms
- C. use of O_2 monitors
- D. all of the above
- E. A and B only

Answer Key

Chapter 1

1-1	98.6°F
1-2	140°F
1-3	–4°F
1-4	100°C
1-5	–17.8°C
1-6	–40°C
1-7	283°K
1-8	323°K
1-9	213°K
1-10	–273°C
1-11	–123°C
1-12	77°C
1-13	32°F
1-14	98.6°F
1-15	–279.4°F
1-16	462°K
1-17	269°K
1-18	200°K
1-19	29.5 in Hg
1-20	1020 cm H_2O
1-21	724 mm Hg
1-22	985 cm H_2O
1-23	1.18 atm

1-24	75 mm Hg
1-25	102 cm H_2O
1-26	5.33 kPa
1-27	9.80 kPa
1-28	82.5 ft H_2O
1-29	94.5 mm Hg
1-30	Decreases, 1842.4 psig
1-31	468 mL
1-32	835 mL
1-33	1.83 L
1-34	152 mm Hg
1-35	171 cm H_2O
1-36	Increases, 56.7°C
1-37	P_{O_2} = 300 mm Hg; P_{N_2} = 450 mm Hg
1-38	P_{He} = 616 mm Hg; P_{O_2} = 154 mm Hg
1-39	P_t = 620 mm Hg; F_{O_2} = 0.13; $\%O_2$ = 13%; F_{CO_2} = 0.065; $\%CO_2$ = 6.5%; F_{N_2} = 0.81; $\%N_2$ = 81%
1-40	760 mm Hg
1-41	0.165 mL O_2/dL blood
1-42	0.24 mL O_2/dL blood
1-43	0.36 mL O_2/dL blood
1-44	0.675 mL O_2/dL blood
1-45	1.8 mL O_2/dL blood

1-46	60% O_2
1-47	60% O_2
1-48	32% O_2
1-49	71% O_2
1-50	69% O_2
1-51	25 : 1
1-52	15 : 1
1-53	8 : 1
1-54	5 : 1
1-55	1.3 : 1
1-56	0.3 : 1
1-57	C
1-58	B
1-59	B
1-60	A
1-61	D
1-62	C
1-63	C
1-64	C
1-65	B
1-66	D
1-67	B

Chapter 2

2-1	423 L, approximately 70 minutes
2-2	14 L, approximately 4.5 minutes
2-3	82 L, approximately 20 minutes
2-4	196 L, approximately 19.5 minutes
2-5	5645 L, approximately 18 hours and 48 minutes
2-6	2509 L, approximately 20 hours and 54 minutes
2-7	747 psig
2-8	1594 psig
2-9	733 psig

2-10	611 psig
2-11	1419 psig
2-12	3 H-cylinders
2-13	62 minutes
2-17	approximately 8 hours and 36 minutes
2-18	117.3 lb
2-19	353 H-cylinders
2-33	C
2-34	A
2-35	C
2-36	C
2-37	B
2-38	D
2-39	B
2-40	C
2-41	E
2-42	B
2-43	E
2-44	A
2-45	C
2-46	B
2-47	D
2-48	D
2-49	D
2-50	D

Chapter 3

3-13	B
3-14	A
3-15	C
3-16	C
3-17	C
3-18	A
3-19	B

3-20	D
3-21	D
3-22	A
3-23	B
3-24	B
3-25	C
3-26	C

4-26	C
4-27	E
4-28	D
4-29	D
4-30	C
4-31	D
4-32	C

Chapter 4

4-1	214 mm Hg, 164 mm Hg
4-2	713 mm Hg, 673 mm Hg
4-3	150 mm Hg, 75 mm Hg
4-4	120 mm Hg, 70 mm Hg
4-5	287 mm Hg, 262 mm Hg
4-6	66 mm Hg, 41 mm Hg
4-7	469 mm Hg, 419 mm Hg
4-8	2233 mm Hg, 2193 mm Hg
4-9	20 Vol%
4-10	18.3 Vol%
4-11	15 Vol%
4-12	20.2 Vol%
4-13	12.2 Vol%
4-14	6.9 Vol%
4-15	14.6 Vol%
4-16	229 mm Hg, 179 mm Hg
4-17	1853 mm Hg, 1813 mm Hg
4-18	70 mm Hg, 20 mm Hg
4-19	133 mm Hg, 83 mm Hg
4-20	603°F
4-21	Increase, 833 mL
4-22	2.86 g/L
4-23	Increases, Increase
4-24	Hb: 17.4 mL of O_2 ; Plasma: 3.3 mL of O_2
4-25	D

Chapter 5

5-1	22 mg/L, approx. 23 mm Hg
5-2	51 mg/L, 55 mm Hg
5-3	21.8 mg/L, 22.3 mm Hg
5-4	5.5 mg/L, approx. 5.3 mm Hg
5-5	22.8 mg/L, approx. 23.5 mm Hg
5-6	160 mm Hg, 600 mm Hg
5-7	155 mm Hg, 582 mm Hg
5-8	148 mm Hg, 557 mm Hg
5-9	239 mm Hg, 359 mm Hg
5-10	246 mm Hg, 369 mm Hg
5-11	155 mm Hg, 581 mm Hg
5-12	1.23 L
5-13	3.40 L
5-14	4.19 L
5-15	1.86 L
5-16	6.55 L
5-17	3.50 L
5-18	6.74 L
5-23	26.6 mg/L
5-24	31.6 mg/L
5-25	43.9 mg/L
5-28	48 L/min
5-29	50 L/min
5-30	60 L/min
5-31	66 L/min
5-32	78 L/min

5-33 36 L/min

5-34 30 L/min

5-35 24 L/min

5-36. Many jet nebulizer jets will only allow 12 to 15 L/min of gas to pass through their jet at a driving pressure of 50 psi. As the FIO_2 setting is increased, the entrainment port becomes smaller and less air is entrained. This results in lower flows to the patient. Nebulizers are available which can generate high flows at high FIO_2 settings.

5-37. Any type of back-pressure results in decreased flows to the patient at a higher FIO_2 because entrainment is decreased. This may result in an unknown concentration of O_2 being delivered to the patient since room air may be inhaled as flows decrease.

5-38. Routinely room air would be the delivery gas to the patient when using a USN. Remove the line from the fan and use some other delivery system to power the USN for aerosol delivery. Some options for delivering 40% oxygen would include an entrainment device, an oxygen blender, or titrating air and oxygen thereby manually blending them together.

5-39. Very little. The FIO_2 should stay at 40%. Unless the increased total flow creates increased downstream back-pressure, the FIO_2 should not be affected by increasing the flow through the entrainment device. The ratio of source gas to entrained gas should remain constant; thus the FIO_2 will not change.

5-40 a. Gas passing through the humidifier is heated and humidified. As the gas travels along the tube, it is cooled. As the gas cools, it reaches its dew point and further cooling results in water condensation. This condensate is what collects in the tubing. Water collection in the tubing is an indication that the gas delivered to the patient is at 100% RH at the temperature delivered to the patient. If no condensation occurs, the delivery gas is at less than 100% RH.

5-40 b. No. This is not an entrainment device. Flow rate and FIO_2 will remain constant.

5-41. *Problem:* The pressure release is activated on the bubble humidifier. Most likely something is obstructing the flow of oxygen out of the humidifier, causing the "pop-off" to vent excess pressure.
Action: Find and relieve the obstruction.

5-42. *Problem:* Probably, there is a leak in the system.
Action: Tighten the connections at the DISS adapter to the flowmeter and tighten the water jar onto the lid.

5-43. Situation 1.
Problem: Water has accumulated in the wide-bore tubing creating increased back-pressure.
Action: Drain the water but not back into the nebulizer. You may want to consider placing a water collection device in-line at the lowest loop of the tubing.

5-43. Situation 2.
Problem: The end of the tube is partially blocked, creating increased back-pressure.
Action: Reposition the tube and cut a V-shaped notch in the end of the tube to prevent this from happening.

5-43. Situation 3.
Problem: The connector is too small and is creating back-pressure in the system.
Action: Find appropriate sized connectors for use with the analyzer and do not use small connectors in such a system.

5-44 B

5-45 D

5-46 D

5-47 C

5-48 D

5-49 B

5-50 B

5-51 D

5-52 C

5-53   A

5-54   A

5-55   C

5-56   A

Chapter 6

6-8.   *Problem*: It is likely that the tongue is obstructing the airway. High pressures are being generated which result in air being forced into the stomach.
Action: Hyperextend the neck some more. Use slow breaths, thus generating a lower upper airway pressure. Ask someone else to perform the Sellick maneuver by placing some pressure on the larynx to collapse the esophagus. This is to prevent air from going into the stomach. The use of an oropharyngeal airway may also be appropriate. If the abdomen is over-distended, the air may need to be removed by gentle pressure on the abdomen or with the use of an N-G tube. There is a danger of the patient vomiting and aspirating while removing this gas.

6-9.   *Problem*: The patient has return of the gag reflex. Maybe he is waking up.
Action: Remove the bite block. Do not tape it in place. Taping the bite block in place may result in vomiting and aspiration.

6-10.   *Problem*: The EOA was probably inserted into the trachea. The gas used for ventilation has no place to go except into the stomach.
Action: It would be best to place a second EOA into the esophagus, then remove the first EOA and ventilate the patient. Removing the EOA first and intubating with an ET tube would increase the chance of aspiration if regurgitation were to occur.

6-11.   *Problem*: Most commonly, this suggests a right main stem intubation. However, absence of breath sounds could also indicate a pneumothorax, obstructed airway, atelectasis, or in rare cases a prior pneumonectomy.

Action: Observe the depth markings on the tube. It is probably inserted further than it should be. Average depth of insertion of an ET tube for a male is 23 cm and for a female 21 cm at the teeth (add 2 cm for nasal intubation). Withdraw the ET tube 2 cm and recheck breath sounds. Repeat if necessary. If moving the tube does not solve the problem, obtain a chest X-ray for confirmation of tube position or other condition.

6-12.   *Problem*: Probably, the cuff was torn during intubation. This makes it impossible to inflate the cuff and develop a seal.
Action: Remove the tube, manually ventilate the patient with a BVM device, and then reintubate with a new tube.

6-13.   *Problem*: The problem could be due to many factors. The light bulb could be loose or burned out. The batteries could be dead or the contacts inside the handle could be loose.
Action: A quick check for a loose bulb can be done, but the patient must be the first priority. Either ventilate the patient with a BVM or obtain another laryngoscope and proceed with the intubation. If no other laryngoscope is available, continue BVM ventilation, or attempt a blind nasal intubation while someone else troubleshoots the problem.

6-14.   *Problem*: Patients who require intubation need the appropriate size ET tube.
Action:
1. Select from a chart listing acceptable sizes based on age or weight.
2. Select a tube approximately the size of the external nares.
3. Select a tube the size of the end of the little finger.
4. Use prior experience to guide selection.

6-15.   *Problem*: Pressure cannot be measured without a manometer, and it should be less than 20 mm Hg.
Action: Although squeezing the pilot balloon is an unacceptable method for determining cuff pressure, a rock-hard pilot balloon suggests that there is too much pressure in the cuff. Suction the posterior oral pharynx as well as you can to remove secretions. Attach a syringe to the pilot balloon

Attach a syringe to the pilot balloon and slowly begin to withdraw volume. Since the patient is on a mechanical ventilator, when the cuff pressure drops low enough, a leak will occur. At this point, inject just enough air to seal the leak. This is the minimal occluding volume technique. If the pilot balloon is still very hard, the minimal leak technique should be used. If secretions entered the trachea from above the cuff, the patient may need to be suctioned. Measure cuff pressure when a manometer is available.

6-16. *Problem:* The tube is too small for the patient, and the cuff is unable to create a seal in the airway at an appropriate pressure.
Action: The tube should be replaced with a larger one. In this situation, the patient may not be at high risk for developing tracheal wall damage. Endotracheal tube cuffs can be inflated to a point where their compliance curve flattens off. That is, a little additional volume creates a large change in pressure. It is assumed that the cuff pressure measured is also the pressure which is exerted against the tracheal wall. If the cuff is not creating a seal in the airway, the cuff may not be exerting excessive pressure against the tracheal wall.

6-17.
1. *Hypoxemia*—hyperoxygenate for 1–2 min prior to suctioning
2. *Atelectasis*—low suction pressure, short time period for suctioning
3. *Arrhythmias*—gentle suctioning, hyperoxygenate
4. *Coughing*—gentle suctioning, instill lidocaine
5. *Vagal stimulation*—gentle suctioning
6. *Contamination*—sterile technique, closed system suctioning
7. *Hypotension*—gentle suctioning, hyperoxygenate, short suction time period
8. *Bronchospasm*—instill lidocaine, use of bronchodilator
9. *Hemoptysis*—low suction pressure, intermittent suction
10. *Increased intracranial pressure*—hyperoxygenate, hyperventilate, use of lidocaine
11. *Mucosal trauma*—low suction pressure, intermittent suction

6-18
(a) 20 FR, 15 FR
(b) 18 FR, 13 FR
(d) 14 FR, 10 FR
(e) 12 FR, 9 FR
(f) 10 FR, 7 FR
(g) 8 FR, 6 FR
(h) 6 FR, 4 FR

6-21 A

6-22 B

6-23 C

6-24 C

6-25 B

6-26 B

6-27 A

6-28 D

6-29 A

6-30 D

6-31 B

6-32 C

6-33 B

6-34 A

6-35 C

6-36 D

6-37 C

6-38 C

6-39 B

Chapter 7

7-9. *Problem:* The one-way inlet valve is leaking or totally missing from the bag. The patient is not being properly ventilated.
Action: The immediate concern is the patient. Ventilate the patient with whatever means is available. When appropriate, disassemble the bag and fix the one-way inlet valve.

7-10. *Problem:* The inlet valve is probably sticking and not opening like it should.
Action: Again the patient must be the first concern. When appropriate, dis-

assemble the bag and free the one-way inlet valve.

7-11. *Problem:* A very low FIO2 is being delivered to the patient.
Action: The flow rate of O2 can be increased, and the bag can be manually restricted so that fill time is prolonged. Try to obtain a reservoir. These factors will help increase the FIO2 delivered.

7-12 D

7-13 C

7-14 B

7-15 A

7-16 A

7-17 A

7-18 E

7-19 D

7-20 E

7-21 B

7-22 D

Chapter 8

8-5 D

8-6 D

8-7 B

8-8 B

8-9 C

8-10 D

8-11 A

8-12 A

8-13 B

8-14 A

8-15 D

8-16 D

8-17 D

8-18 A

8-19 E

8-20 D

8-21 D

8-22 E

8-23 B

8-24 A

8-25 D

8-26 D

8-27 C

8-28 C

8-29 B

Chapter 9

9-2. 40%. Since it reads a dry sample, it will read the same regardless of its placement in the circuit. Perform an experiment to test this phenomenon.

9-3. The reading proximal to the humidifier will be 40%, whereas the reading distal to the humidifier will be less. This is because humidity must now be considered. The actual reading can be computed by performing the following calculations.
  • proximal:
   760 mm Hg $\times.4 = 304$ mm Hg (PO2)
  • distal:
   $(760 - 47) \times.4 = 285$ mm Hg
(285 represents 40% of 713. However, 285 is actually part of the total pressure, so when compared to the total pressure it is $285/760 =.375$ or 37.5% O2.)
Perform an experiment to test this.

9-4. 1. Maybe the individual accuracy and linearity of the devices are at fault.
2. Some sensors may be reading a wet sample compared to a dry sample.
3. It may be due to random error, yet falling within the acceptable limits of variability of 2 to 3% as given by the manufacturer.

9-5. *Answer:* Possible actions would include:
1. Make sure the nebulizer is set at 40%.
2. Recalibrate the analyzer and reanalyze.
3. Make sure there is no downstream obstruction creating back pressure in the system.
4. Check the FIO_2 with another analyzer. If the second analyzer also reads 50%, then the problem is most likely with the nebulizer, and it is delivering 50% even though it is set at 40%. It would be best to replace the nebulizer. If the second analyzer reads 40%, it is more likely that the first analyzer is inaccurate.

9-6. *Answer:* Since the positive pressure affects the partial pressure of the O_2 in the gas sample, the PO_2 will be increased and the O_2 analyzer will record an increased FIO_2 reading. The following steps can be used to compute the value:
1. Convert cm H_2O to mm Hg, 60 cm H_2O = 44 mm Hg.
2. Then add the system pressure to the atmospheric pressure—760 + 44 = 804 mm Hg—the total pressure in the system.
3. Multiply the total (dry) pressure by 0.6—804 × .6 = 482.
4. Since the analyzer was calibrated at 760 mm Hg, the 482 is divided by 760 to determine the FIO_2 which will be expressed by the analyzer—482/760 = 63.5%. This occurs under dry conditions.
Perform an experiment to confirm this.

9-8. Oximetry was not a valid assessment tool. It represents an inaccurate and worthless value which lulls the caregiver into a false sense of security. A blood gas with co-oximetry must be performed. Co-oximetry, not to be confused with oximetry, actually measures the COHb level. Once the COHb levels are known, appropriate therapy can be continued. *Note:* This same phenomenon can occur with individuals who smoke. COHb levels of smokers can easily reach levels up to 12%. O_2 Sat readings via pulse oximetry would be falsely elevated in these individuals.

9-9. The O_2 Sat reading is lower than what would be expected for a PaO_2 of 80 mm Hg. The patient may have a shift to the right of the O_2Hb dissociation curve which would explain this situation. Alternatively, it could indicate that the pulse oximeter is within its range of acceptable limits of accuracy, but the patient actually has a saturation of 96%. Further, it could suggest that the pulse oximetry is just inaccurate.

9-10. The $PaCO_2$ level is elevated. This may be due to increased CO_2 production with normal ventilation, or due to decreased alveolar ventilation. This is common in the COPD patient.

9-11. The patient attempted an inspiration in the middle of exhalation.

9-12. Airway obstruction and incomplete exhalation

9-13. Rapid respiratory rate, hyperventilation or possible increased VD/VT.

9-14 C

9-15 D

9-16 B

9-17 B

9-18 B

9-19 B

9-20 A

9-21 D

9-22 D

9-23 C

9-24 B

9-25 C

9-26 B

9-27 A

9-28 B

9-29 D

9-30 D

Chapter 10

10-3	C
10-4	B
10-5	A
10-6	D
10-7	C
10-8	D
10-9	C
10-10	B
10-11	A
10-12	D
10-13	C
10-14	D
10-15	D

Chapter 11

11-1	B
11-2	C
11-3	A
11-4	B
11-5	C
11-6	A
11-7	E
11-8	D
11-9	D
11-10	E

Chapter 12

12-1. Some patients may exert what seems to be a good effort but are unable or unwilling to take deep breaths. In this case the patient is taking deep breaths (good chest expansion), but it is not registering on the device. Encourage the patient to keep his lips tight and/or use a nose clip to ensure that inhaled air passes through the device. This may not improve the actual therapy, but it allows the documentation of the volume.

12-2. The machine is probably functioning properly but some of the settings need to be adjusted. The patient is creating a large negative pressure of −10 cm H_2O because the sensitivity control is not set properly. Increase the machine sensitivity by moving the magnet further away from the metal plate until only −1 to −2 cm H_2O is needed to initiate inspiration. The second situation in which the needle remains at a low pressure during the breath is due to the patient actively inhaling during the treatment. Encourage the patient to relax following the initiation of the breath or increase the flow rate to better meet the patient's spontaneous inspiratory flow.

12-3. The pressure limit is being reached rapidly with every breath. Probably, the patient is obstructing the mouth piece with his tongue or maintaining a closed glottis. Encourage the patient to avoid this. Extremely high flow rates or patient coughing may also result in a similar situation.

12-5. There are three reasons why the FIO_2 is higher than 40%.
1. The venturi has a gate (a spring loaded valve) that closes when the pressure reaches approximately 12–15 cm H_2O. Little mixed gas enters the pressurized system after that point.
2. Although the gate closes, the venturi is still supplied with 100% O_2. This gas is "dumped" into the ambient chamber of the device and is entrained with the next breath. This results in an increased FIO_2 coming through the venturi on the next breath.
3. Once the venturi gate closes, the system still receives gas flow through the nebulizer line. This gas is 100% O_2 and is responsible for completing the inspiration to the desired pressure.

12-7	D
12-8	A

12-9	B
12-10	C
12-11	C
12-12	D
12-13	E
12-14	D
12-15	B
12-16	E
12-17	E
12-18	A
12-19	D

Chapter 13

13-4	A
13-5	E
13-6	D
13-7	D
13-8	D
13-9	D
13-10	D
13-11	E
13-12	D
13-13	A
13-14	D
13-15	A
13-16	E
13-17	D
13-18	D
13-19	D
13-20	B
13-21	C
13-22	A
13-23	B
13-24	C
13-24	B

13-26	D
13-27	D
13-28	B

Chapter 14

14-9	D
14-10	D
14-11	D
14-12	A
14-13	B
14-14	A
14-15	B
14-16	D
14-17	B
14-18	D
14-19	D
14-20	C
14-21	B
14-22	B
14-23	A
14-24	B
14-25	B
14-26	B
14-27	E
14-28	D

Chapter 15

15-3	D
15-4	E
15-5	A
15-6	E
15-7	C
15-8	D
15-9	B

15-10 A
15-11 B
15-12 B

Chapter 16

16-2   B
16-3   C
16-4   D
16-5   D
16-6   A
16-7   D
16-8   D
16-9   B
16-10 D
16-11 A
16-12 D

Chapter 17

17-2   E
17-3   A
17-4   D
17-5   E
17-6   D
17-7   C
17-8   D
17-9   D
17-10 E
17-11 D
17-12 C

Chapter 18

18-7   B

18-8   D
18-9   D
18-10 E
18-11 B
18-12 D
18-13 E
18-14 C
18-15 C
18-16 A
18-17 D

Chapter 19

19-2   A
19-3   B
19-4   A
19-5   C
19-6   D
19-7   B

Chapter 20

20-1   A
20-2   D
20-3   D
20-4   B
20-5   D
20-6   C
20-7   D
20-8   D
20-9   B
20-10 C
20-11 D
20-12 E
20-13 C
20-14 B

20-15	C		21-9	D
20-16	C		21-10	C
20-17	B		21-11	C
20-18	A		21-12	B
20-19	B		21-13	D
20-20	D		21-14	D
20-21	C		21-15	D
20-22	A			
20-23	D			

Chapter 22

22-1	D
22-2	C

Chapter 21

22-3	A
22-4	D

21-1	B	
21-2	D	
21-3	E	
21-4	D	
21-5	A	
21-6	E	
21-7	D	
21-8	D	

22-5	B
22-6	A
22-7	C
22-8	D
22-9	C
22-10	D